# Practice Test #1

## Practice Questions

1. Which of the following statements is true regarding hypertension and the geriatric patient?
    a. The incidence of hypertension decreases with advancing age.
    b. Individuals with a systolic blood pressure of > 160 mm Hg and a diastolic blood pressure of 100 mm Hg are considered hypertensive.
    c. Female gender is a risk factor for hypertension.
    d. Headache, disorientation, confusion, and epistaxis may be indicative of hypertension.

2. An elderly patient is admitted to a medical-surgical unit with a diagnosis of hypertension. After several hours on the unit, the patient's blood pressure is noted to be 210/140 mm Hg and a diagnosis of hypertensive crisis is made. Upon review of the patient's medical history, it is noted that she has never been treated for hypertension. Which of the following treatment strategies is **not** appropriate to consider?
    a. Sublingual nifedipine should be administered to rapidly lower the patient's blood pressure to prevent organ damage.
    b. The patient's blood pressure should be lowered over a period of hours to days to decrease the risk of cerebral and myocardial ischemia.
    c. Antihypertensive therapy should be initiated along with the establishment of a blood pressure reduction goal clinically appropriate for the patient.
    d. Nonpharmacologic treatment options such as providing a quiet environment for the patient to rest should also be utilized.

3. You are providing education to a 70-year-old patient recently diagnosed with hyperlipidemia. Which of the following statements by the patient indicates a need for further education?
    a. "I should reduce my intake of egg yolks and organ meats."
    b. "I need to report new or worsening muscle aches to my doctor if I experience them while taking my Lipitor."
    c. "My goal is to decrease my HDL level from 60 to 40."
    d. "I should limit my intake of grapefruit or grapefruit juice while on my Lipitor."

4. A 68-year-old patient with a history of myocardial infarction and renal failure is admitted with a diagnosis of chest pain. The registered nurse caring for the patient alerts you that the patient has increasing shortness of breath, is tachypneic and cyanotic, and has had an acute mental status change. Vital signs are BP 70/30, HR 160, and RR 42. The patient's peripheral pulses are barely palpable. Which of the following conditions are you concerned the patient may be experiencing?
    a. myocardial infarction
    b. cardiac tamponade
    c. endocarditis
    d. pulmonary edema

5. Which of the following statements is **not** true regarding acute coronary syndrome (ACS)?
    a. ACS includes both unstable angina and myocardial infarction (MI).
    b. Age is a strong predictor of outcome in ACS.
    c. Elderly ACS patients are less likely to receive evidenced-based interventions including revascularization therapy and the use of cardiovascular medications.
    d. Medical advances in the treatment of ACS that have been shown to decrease mortality and increase life expectancy have primarily been aimed at adults 65 years and older.

6. A 78-year-old patient arrives for her appointment with her primary care physician. She presents with a cough and dyspnea, and is complaining of extreme fatigue. Her vital signs are BP 88/40, HR 130, RR 36. A diagnosis of acute decompensated heart failure is made and the patient is transported to the hospital and admitted. Which of the following treatment options would **not** be appropriate for this patient?
    a. diuretic therapy
    b. supplemental oxygen
    c. administration of morphine sulfate
    d. sodium restriction

7. Which of the following statements is **not** true regarding the physiologic cardiac changes that occur with aging?
    a. systemic vascular resistance is decreased
    b. the myocardium stiffens and becomes more rigid with age
    c. the myocardium is less sensitive to catecholamines
    d. increased afterload on the left ventricle

8. Which of the following organisms is associated with the highest mortality rate in patients with endocarditis?
    a. *Escherichia coli*
    b. *Staphylococcus aureus*
    c. *Klebsiella pneumoniae*
    d. *Proteus vulgaris*

9. All of the following statements are true regarding cardiogenic shock with the exception of which statement?
    a. Myocardial infarction with failure of the left ventricle is the most common cause of cardiogenic shock.
    b. Cardiogenic shock is more common in non-ST elevation MI patients
    c. Symptoms of hypoperfusion associated with cardiogenic shock may include decreased urinary output and mental status changes.
    d. The diagnosis of cardiogenic shock is often made through pulmonary artery catheterization.

10. Which of the following conditions may contribute to the development of cardiogenic pulmonary edema?
    a. left ventricular diastolic dysfunction
    b. left ventricular systolic dysfunction
    c. new-onset rapid atrial fibrillation
    d. myocardial infarction
    e. all of the above

11. A 64-year-old patient is admitted to the telemetry unit with a diagnosis of new-onset atrial fibrillation. A workup is conducted and the patient does not have evidence of underlying heart disease. Which of the following noncardiac conditions in the patient's history may be a contributing factor in his diagnosis of atrial fibrillation?
   a. hyperthyroidism
   b. rheumatoid arthritis
   c. chronic kidney disease
   d. hiatal hernia
   e. all of the above

12 Which of the following is a clinical predictor of increased stroke risk in patients with asymptomatic carotid artery stenosis?
   a. female gender
   b. history of smoking
   c. poorly controlled hypertension
   d. bradycardia

13. Which of the following "P" symptoms associated with acute arterial insufficiency is incorrect?
   a. pain
   b. pallor
   c. pulselessness
   d. peripheral neuropathy

14. The type of cardiomyopathy characterized by reduced diastolic volume of either or both ventricles with normal or near-normal systolic function and wall thickness is known as:
   a. hypertrophic cardiomyopathy
   b. restrictive cardiomyopathy
   c. dilated cardiomyopathy
   d. idiopathic cardiomyopathy

15. Which of the following congenital heart defects involves the malformation of the tricuspid valve, which causes blood to leak back into the right atrium and may not be diagnosed until adulthood?
   a. Ebstein's anomaly
   b. atrial septal defect
   c. coarctation of the aorta
   d. patent ductus arteriosus

16. A 70-year-old female patient in the cardiovascular intensive care unit is recovering from a coronary artery bypass graft. She has a history of hypertension and severely narrowed coronary arteries. Given the patient's history, which complication is she at an increased risk of developing postoperatively?
   a. aortic dissection
   b. pleural effusion
   c. phrenic nerve damage
   d. thrombocytopenia

17. Which of the following statements is **not** true regarding blunt cardiac injury in the adult patient?
    a. Blunt cardiac injuries are often associated with other thoracic injuries including rib fractures and pneumothorax.
    b. The majority of patients with blunt cardiac injury are asymptomatic
    c. Coronary artery injuries are the most common type of blunt cardiac injury.
    d. More severe blunt cardiac injuries may lead to exsanguination, pericardial tamponade, and death.

18. All of the following are considerations in increasing the risk of bleeding associated with antithrombotic therapy in elderly patients except?
    a. poly-pharmacy resulting in drug-drug interactions
    b. increased clotting
    c. increased fibrinolysis
    d. decreased renal function

19. Which of the following statements is true regarding penetrating chest trauma?
    a. Penetrating chest trauma is more common than blunt chest trauma.
    b. Penetration of the thoracic wall most commonly occurs from industrial type accidents.
    c. Most penetrating chest injuries require major surgical intervention.
    d. Pneumothorax should be suspected in any patient with penetrating chest trauma.

20. A 70-year-old patient with chronic kidney disease is admitted to a medical-surgical unit with shortness of breath, fatigue, and bilateral ankle edema. The patient has a history of type 2 diabetes and was recently started on a dipeptidyl peptidase-4 (DPP-4) inhibitor (saxagliptin). You know that the FDA recently issued a MedWatch safety alert for patients taking DPP-4 inhibitors that contain saxagliptin and alogliptin. Which of the following statements is true regarding DPP-4 inhibitors containing saxagliptin and alogliptin?
    a. Health care professionals should consider discontinuing medications containing saxagliptin and alogliptin in patients who develop heart failure and should monitor their diabetes control.
    b. Shortness of breath, fatigue, and swelling are all commonly experienced symptoms in patients taking DPP-4 inhibitors.
    c. If patients experience shortness of breath, fatigue, weight gain, and/or swelling, they should immediately discontinue the DPP-4 inhibitor.
    d. DPP-4 inhibitors containing saxagliptin and alogliptin are not FDA approved for the treatment of type 2 diabetes.

21. Which type of pulmonary embolism lodges at the bifurcation of the main pulmonary artery and extends into the left and right pulmonary arteries?
    a. segmental
    b. sub-segmental
    c. saddle
    d. hemodynamically stable

22. A 60-year-old patient arrives at the emergency department with shortness of breath and mental status changes. Vital signs are BP 80/44, HR 120, RR 36, pulse oximetry 90% on 3 L of oxygen. Diagnostic testing confirms the diagnosis of a pulmonary embolism. Repeat vital signs 15 minutes later are BP 74/40, HR 124, RR 32. Which of the following first-line treatment options is the best choice?
    a. administration of vasopressors
    b. intravenous fluid resuscitation
    c. placement of an inferior vena cava filter
    d. embolectomy

23. Which of the following clinical findings may be seen on chest radiograph for a patient with a suspected pulmonary embolism?
    a. atelectasis
    b. normal chest radiograph
    c. cardiomegaly
    d. all of the above

24. Which of the following diagnostic tests would be most appropriate to utilize to differentiate asthma from other respiratory illnesses such as chronic obstructive pulmonary disease?
    a. chest x-ray
    b. pulmonary function tests
    c. electrocardiography
    d. computed tomography scan of chest

25. You are seeing a 72-year-old patient in your primary care office. The patient was diagnosed with asthma 1 year ago and is now presenting with wheezing, chest tightness, and cough. Upon interviewing the patient, she mentions that she recently started a "few new medications." Which of the following new medications that the patient is taking may be contributing to the exacerbation of her asthma symptoms?
    a. lisinopril
    b. doxepin
    c. pantoprazole
    d. losartan

26. You are performing a history and physical on a 70-year-old patient who is experiencing dyspnea on exertion. The patient states that in addition to her shortness of breath, she has been experiencing heart palpitations, fatigue, and an intolerance to heat. Which of the following potential diagnoses could be a contributing factor in the patient's dyspnea?
    a. anemia
    b. psychogenic dyspnea
    c. aortic stenosis
    d. thyroid disease

27. The World Health Organization (WHO) classifies patients with pulmonary hypertension (PH) into 5 groups based upon etiology. Patients in group 1 have which of the following types of pulmonary hypertension?
    a. patients with pulmonary hypertension secondary to hypoxemia
    b. patients with pulmonary hypertension secondary to left-sided heart disease
    c. patients with idiopathic arterial hypertension
    d. patients with pulmonary hypertension secondary to thromboembolic occlusion of the pulmonary vasculature

28. The most common risk factor for obstructive sleep apnea is:
    a. male gender
    b. obesity
    c. smoking
    d. craniofacial abnormalities

29. You are rounding on a medical surgical unit and are seeing a 74-year-old male patient who was recently diagnosed with aspiration pneumonia. An anaerobic bacterium is the suspected pathogen. Which of the following treatment options would you **not** consider?
    a. clindamycin
    b. amoxicillin-clavulanate
    c. metronidazole plus amoxicillin
    d. moxifloxacin

30. The most common site of aspiration of foreign bodies is the:
    a. right main stem bronchus
    b. oropharynx
    c. trachea
    d. left main stem bronchus

31. Which of the following is an indication for lung volume reduction surgery for a patient with emphysema?
    a. age 65 years and younger
    b. longer than 12 months of smoking cessation
    c. inability to complete a 6- to 10-week pulmonary rehabilitation program
    d. marked airflow obstruction on spirometry

32. Which of the following is a treatment-related predictor of mortality in acute respiratory distress syndrome (ARDS)?
    a. negative fluid balance
    b. early intubation
    c. platelet transfusion
    d. treatment with glucocorticoids prior to development of ARDS

33. Pulmonary interstitial emphysema is most likely to occur in patients with which condition?
    a. interstitial pneumonia
    b. chronic obstructive pulmonary disease
    c. non-small cell lung cancer
    d. prior intubation/mechanical ventilation

34. You are working in the emergency department when a 60-year-old patient arrives after a motor vehicle accident. The patient experienced blunt thoracic trauma as a result of the accident and undergoes a CT scan of the chest. A diagnosis of occult pneumothorax (6 mm in length) is made based on the CT scan results. The patient is hemodynamically stable and is not experiencing any type of respiratory distress or compromise. Which of the following treatment options is most appropriate for this patient?
 a. placement of chest tube
 b. observation
 c. positive pressure ventilation
 d. surgical thoracotomy

35. Which of the following anatomic changes would you expect for a patient who has undergone a pneumonectomy?
 a. rapid accumulation of fluid into the post-pneumonectomy space
 b. obliteration of the post-pneumonectomy space
 c. shifting of the mediastinum away from the post-pneumonectomy space
 d. elevation of the hemidiaphragm

36. Which of the following conditions develops in patients with chronic obstructive pulmonary disease and causes development of cyanosis?
 a. cor pulmonale
 b. secondary polycythemia
 c. fibrosis
 d. mucous hypersecretion

37. Which of the following familial/congenital conditions is not associated with the development of central diabetes insipidus (CDI)?
 a. Wolfram syndrome
 b. congenital hypopituitarism
 c. familial central diabetes insipidus
 d. Bartter syndrome

38. Which of the following medications **not** used in the treatment of diabetes has the potential to cause hypoglycemia?
 a. beta-blockers
 b. estrogens
 c. sympathomimetics
 d. phenothiazines

39. The recommended first step in the treatment of diabetic ketoacidosis and hyperglycemic hyperosmolar state is:
 a. administration of IV insulin analogues
 b. administration of potassium replacement
 c. administration of sodium bicarbonate
 d. infusion of isotonic saline

40. Which of the following is **not** a first-line treatment option for a patient experiencing thyroid storm?
    a. administration of a beta-blocker
    b. administration of an iodine solution
    c. administration of a glucocorticoid
    d. plasmapheresis

41. According to the American Diabetes Association (ADA) and European Association for the Study of Diabetes (EASD) consensus guideline for pharmacotherapy to control hyperglycemia in type 2 diabetes, the addition of a secondary medication is recommended when which of the following conditions occur?
    a. Treatment goal of hemoglobin A1c < 7% with metformin and lifestyle intervention is not achieved within 3 months.
    b. Treatment goal of hemoglobin A1c < 7% with metformin and lifestyle intervention is not achieved within 6 months.
    c. Treatment goal of hemoglobin A1c < 7% with metformin and lifestyle intervention is not achieved within 12 months.
    d. Treatment goal of hemoglobin A1c < 7% with metformin and lifestyle intervention is not achieved within 18 months.

42. Which of the following agents is **not** recommended in the treatment of type 2 diabetes?
    a. thiazolidinediones
    b. sulfonylureas
    c. bromocriptine
    d. DPP-4 inhibitor

43. Which of the following statements regarding the rate of correction of hyponatremia in patients with syndrome of inappropriate antidiuretic hormone secretion (SIADH) is **not** correct?
    a. Patients with severe neurologic symptoms require a slow correction of hyponatremia.
    b. Treatment of patients with asymptomatic hyponatremia should focus on the underlying cause and may only be treated with fluid restriction (if cause cannot be
    c. Patients with mild neurologic symptoms may be treated with fluid restriction and oral salt tablets.
    d. Fluid restriction (fluid intake goal of < 800 mL/day) is a standard treatment option for most patients with SIADH.

44. Which of the following joints is the most commonly affected in septic arthritis?
    a. hip
    b. knee
    c. wrist
    d. ankle

45. You are rounding on a 74-year-old patient with suspected rhabdomyolysis. Which of the following items in the patient's history and physical may be the cause?
    a. chronic alcohol abuse
    b. renal failure
    c. patient is currently taking a statin
    d. patient is currently taking a beta blocker
    e. all of the above
    f. a and c

46. What is the most common type of functional movement disorder?
    a. myoclonus
    b. dystonia
    c. functional tremor
    d. functional gait disorder

47. Which of the following is **not** considered a possible manifestation of a gait disorder?
    a. dragging gait
    b. knee buckling
    c. swaying gait
    d. cautious gait

48. The leading cause of death from injury in men and women older than 65 years is:
    a. motor vehicle accident
    b. falls
    c. fire
    d. suffocation

49. You are rounding on a 62-year-old male patient who was admitted to the medical surgical unit after a fall off of a ladder that resulted in a femur fracture. When assessing the patient you note that the patient is complaining of intense pain and decreased sensation and paresthesia in the fractured leg. You assess the affected leg and find firmness, swelling, and tightness. Which of the following conditions do you suspect the patient might be experiencing?
    a. compartment syndrome
    b. osteomyelitis
    c. fat embolism
    d. deep vein thrombosis

50. The diagnosis of compartment syndrome is made by physical assessment and _____.
    a. diagnostic x-ray
    b. CT scan
    c. serum creatine kinase
    d. the measurement of intracompartmental pressures

51. A 62-year-old male patient diagnosed with stage 3 small cell lung cancer is admitted to the oncology floor with increased somnolence, weakness, nausea and vomiting, and diffuse abdominal pain. His wife reports he has become increasingly weak over the past 3 days and has exhibited a change in mental status. She reports he has not had a bowel movement in 5 days and has been complaining of abdominal pain. Which of the following oncologic complications is a likely explanation for the patient's clinical presentation?
    a. superior vena cava syndrome
    b. septic shock
    c. metastasis to the liver
    d. hypercalcemia

52. Which of the following could be utilized as a preventive strategy in the management of cancer related pain?
    a. Instruct the patient to only take prescribed analgesics when their pain level is moderate to severe to prevent narcotic dependency.
    b. The use of bone-modifying agents to prevent skeletal events including fractures and bone pain caused by bone metastases.
    c. Avoid the use of adjuvant agents or co-analgesics.
    d. The pharmacologic management of pain should begin with mild opioids.

53. Anemia is considered microcytic when the mean corpuscular volume (MCV) is less than _____ fL (femtoliters).
    a. 90 fL
    b. 100 fL
    c. 80 fL
    d. 110 fL

54. Macrocytosis may occur in which of the following disorders?
    a. myelodysplastic syndrome (MDS)
    b. hyperthyroidism
    c. anemia of inflammation
    d. thalassemia

55. Which of the following is **not** a modifiable risk factor associated with over-anticoagulation in the use of warfarin?
    a. medication interactions
    b. acute illness
    c. variations in vitamin K intake
    d. hypotension

56. In patients with thrombocytopenia, the likelihood of severe spontaneous bleeding is associated with platelet counts of _____ or less.
    a. 20,000
    b. 10,000
    c. 50,000
    d. 35,000

57. A 58-year-old female patient is admitted to the medical surgical unit with complaints of extreme fatigue, abdominal pain, and dyspnea. She also reports that she is experiencing pink-tinged urine. Her complete blood cell count results show that she is anemic with an increased reticulocyte count, lactate dehydrogenase (LDH), and bilirubin level. Urinalysis reveals hemoglobinuria with a positive dipstick for heme and negative sediment for red blood cells. Which of the following disorders do you suspect the patient may be diagnosed with?
    a. primary myelofibrosis
    b. myelodysplastic syndrome
    c. hematuria
    d. paroxysmal nocturnal hemoglobinuria (PNH)

58. A 60-year-old patient is admitted to the medical surgical unit with a new diagnosis of limited cutaneous systemic sclerosis. Clinical symptoms of limited cutaneous systemic sclerosis may include CREST syndrome. What does the "T" in CREST syndrome represent?
    a. thrombocytopenia
    b. telangiectasia
    c. tendonitis
    d. thalassemia

59. You are rounding on a 55-year-old female patient with rheumatoid arthritis. She presented to the emergency department with a reddened rash on her arms and legs that was diagnosed as vasculitis. In addition, she complains of pain and tenderness of the face (near the salivary glands). Which of the following conditions might this patient be experiencing?
    a. osteonecrosis of the jaw
    b. Lyme disease
    c. polymyalgia rheumatica
    d. secondary Sjögren syndrome

60. You are preparing to provide discharge instructions to a 62-year-old female patient recently diagnosed with systemic lupus erythematosus. Which of the following statements would you include in her discharge instructions?
    a. "Avoid exposure to ultraviolet light as it may exacerbate your symptoms"
    b. "You should take a daily vitamin supplement."
    c. "Make sure that your vaccinations are up to date and if not previous immunized, obtain the measles, mumps, and rubella vaccine."
    d. "You can continue taking your herbal supplements."

61. Which of the following statements is true regarding brain arteriovenous malformations (AVM)?
    a. Intracranial hemorrhage is more common in adult patients with brain AVMs.
    b. Focal neurologic deficit is a common presentation in cerebral AVMs.
    c. Patients with cortically located, large, multiple, and superficial-draining AVMs are more likely to present with seizures.
    d. Brain AVM's most commonly present between the ages of 35 to 60 years.

62. Which of the following is **not** a physiologic musculoskeletal change associated with aging?
    a. increased curvature of the spine (kyphosis)
    b. increased fluid in intervertebral disks
    c. decreased tissue elasticity
    d. decreased bone calcium

63. Which of the following statement is **not** true regarding partial (focal) seizures?
    a. Partial (focal) seizures occur in only one hemisphere of the brain.
    b. Partial (focal) seizures can be complex or simple.
    c. Loss of consciousness is associated with complex partial seizures.
    d. The drugs of choice in the treatment of partial (focal) simple seizures are valproic acid and clonazepam.

64. Which of the following types of dementia is associated with early symptoms resembling Parkinson disease?
    a. Lewy body dementia
    b. frontotemporal dementia
    c. vascular dementia
    d. Alzheimer disease

65. Which of the following functional impairments is defined as the inability to recognize objects?
    a. apraxia
    b. agnosia
    c. anomia
    d. anhedonia

66. Which of the following is the most common cause of subarachnoid hemorrhage?
    a. thrombus formation in a cerebral artery
    b. hypertension
    c. rupture of arterial aneurysms
    d. vascular malformations

67. Which of the following is the most common cause of acute toxic-metabolic encephalopathy?
    a. hyponatremia
    b. hypoxia
    c. increased ammonia level
    d. sepsis

68. Normal intracranial pressure in adults is:
    a. < 15 mm Hg
    b. < 20 mm Hg
    c. < 10 mm Hg
    d. < 25 mm Hg

69. Which of the following is **not** considered a reasonable option for monitoring intracranial pressure?
    a. epidural monitors
    b. intra-ventricular monitoring
    c. tissue resonance analysis
    d. fiber optic Camino system

70. Which of the following neurologic conditions would the administration of glucocorticoids be appropriate as a treatment option for?
    a. intracranial hemorrhage
    b intracranial hypertension associated with a brain tumor
    c. increased intracranial pressure
    d. cerebral infarction

71. Flaccid paralysis followed by encephalitis and the presence of a maculopapular rash are indicative of which type of viral infection?
    a. mumps encephalitis
    b. encephalitic rabies
    c. varicella zoster virus
    d. West Nile virus

72. Headaches are a common symptom associated with brain tumors; however, headache is infrequently seen independent of other symptoms. Which of the following are common symptoms associated with headache in patients diagnosed with a brain tumor?
    a. seizures
    b. fatigue
    c. cognitive dysfunction
    d. all of the above

73. Which of the following is the most common form of motor neuron disease?
    a. multiple sclerosis (MS)
    b. amyotrophic lateral sclerosis (ALS)
    c. acute transverse myelitis (TM)
    d. muscular dystrophy

74. The severity of cord syndromes associated with traumatic spinal cord injuries are classified using the American Spinal Injury Association (ASIA) Scale. Which of the following is **not** a classification associated with the ASIA scale?
    a. complete cord injury
    b. sensory incomplete
    c. motor complete
    d. normal

75. Which of the following clinical symptoms is not considered to be exclusion criteria for the administration of recombinant tissue plasminogen activator in the treatment of acute ischemic stroke?
    a. active internal bleeding
    b. serum glucose < 70 mg/dL
    c. symptoms suggestive of subarachnoid hemorrhage
    d. persistent blood pressure elevation (SBP > 185 mm Hg or DBP > 110mm Hg)

76. Which of the following is **not** true regarding patients with a diagnosis of functional gallbladder disorder?
    a. functional gallbladder disease is defined as a motility disorder of the gallbladder
    b. patients typically present with biliary colic
    c. liver and pancreas lab tests are typically abnormal
    d. patients with functional gallbladder disorder are candidates for cholecystectomy if biliary colic and a gallbladder ejection fraction of < 40% is present

77. According to the Rome III criteria, which of the following is **not** a defining symptom of dyspepsia?
    a. early satiation
    b. epigastric pain
    c. weight loss
    d. postprandial fullness

78. Which of the following factors may decrease the risk of colorectal cancer?
    a. increased calcium intake
    b. use of nonsteroidal anti-inflammatory agents
    c. use of aspirin
    d. all of the above

79. Vomiting of food eaten several hours earlier and the presence of a sloshing sound on abdominal auscultation while the patient is moving (succussion splash) may indicate which type of gastrointestinal disorder associated with nausea and vomiting?
    a. cholelithiasis
    b. intestinal obstruction
    c. gastroparesis
    d. acute viral gastroenteritis

80. Which of the following classes of medications has been deemed the most useful as an antiemetic used for chemotherapy induced emesis?
    a. benzamides
    b. 5-HT$_3$ receptor antagonists
    c. butyrophenones
    d. neurokinin receptor antagonists

81. Which of the following is a relatively common side effect of phenothiazines (used in the treatment of nausea and vomiting)?
    a. headache
    b. hypertension
    c. abdominal pain
    d. extrapyramidal reactions

82. Emesis, retching, or coughing prior to hematemesis is indicative of which potential cause of an upper gastrointestinal bleed?
    a. Mallory-Weiss tear
    b. malignancy
    c. peptic ulcer
    d. esophageal ulcer

83. Acute liver failure is diagnosed by all of the following criteria within the exception of _____?
    a. hepatic encephalopathy
    b. elevated aminotransferase levels
    c. elevated platelet count
    d. prolonged prothrombin time

84. Which solid organs are the most commonly injured in blunt abdominal trauma?
    a. pancreas and bowel
    b. diaphragm and stomach
    c. kidneys and bladder
    d. spleen and liver

85. Which of the following statements is true regarding acute hepatitis C infection?
    a. Most patients with acute hepatitis C infection present with right upper quadrant abdominal pain.
    b. Acute illness usually lasts for 2 to 4 weeks.
    c. Patients with acute hepatitis C infection typically have serum aminotransferase levels that are moderately to highly elevated.
    d. Fulminant hepatic failure is a common complication in patients with acute hepatitis C infection.

86. What is the most common risk factor for hepatitis A infection in the United States?
    a. international travel
    b. sexual contact with an infected partner
    c. drug use by injection
    d. food or waterborne exposure

87. The 4 primary clinical findings that characterize chronic pancreatitis include diabetes mellitus, pancreatic calculi, pain, and which other finding?
    a. unexplained anemia
    b. dyspepsia
    c. steatorrhea
    d. diarrhea

88. Muscle and fat mass depletion are associated with which abdominal condition?
    a. inflammatory bowel disease
    b. cholelithiasis
    c. gastroesophageal reflux
    d. hepatitis

89. Which of the following classifications of medications is associated with diverticular perforation?
    a. antispasmodics
    b. selective serotonin uptake inhibitors
    c. beta-blockers
    d. nonsteroidal anti-inflammatory agents

90. The initial medication of choice in the treatment of non-severe *C. difficile* infection is:
    a. vancomycin
    b. fidaxomicin
    c. metronidazole
    d. rifaximin

91. Which of the following is the preferred fluid choice in the treatment of volume depletion of patients with acute kidney injury?
    a. dextrose 5% in water
    b. isotonic saline
    c. Hespan
    d. lactated Ringer's

92. Evidence of kidney damage or decreased kidney function for a period of _____ or more months distinguishes chronic kidney disease from acute kidney injury.
    a. 1 month
    b. 3 months
    c. 6 months
    d. 12 months

93. Overflow incontinence in women is caused by underactivity of the detrusor muscle and _____.
    a. intrinsic sphincteric deficiency
    b. overactive bladder
    c. urethral hypermobility
    d. bladder outlet obstruction

94. Which of the following organisms is most commonly associated with catheter-associated urinary tract infections?
    a. *Pseudomonas aeruginosa*
    b. *Klebsiella pneumoniae*
    c. *Escherichia coli*
    d. *Staphylococcus aureus*

95. Which of the following beverages is associated with a decreased risk of kidney stone formation?
    a. cranberry juice
    b. cola
    c. orange juice
    d. Gatorade

96. Which of the following is **not** a typical presenting symptom in patients with suspected pelvic inflammatory disease?
    a. menorrhagia
    b. purulent endocervical discharge
    c. lower abdominal pain
    d. right upper quadrant pain with referred right shoulder pain

97. Which of the following sexually transmitted infections should be screened for in female patients younger than 25 years annually?
    a. *Chlamydia trachomatis*
    b. syphilis
    c. human immunodeficiency virus (HIV)
    d. *Mycoplasma genitalium*

98. You are rounding on a 74-year-old male patient admitted to the hospital with a diagnosis of mental status change, weakness, constipation, and oliguria. His past medical history includes cirrhosis of the liver and alcoholism. Physical examination reveals a positive Trousseau sign. Which of the following electrolyte abnormalities is this patient experiencing?
   a. hypophosphatemia
   b. hypokalemia
   c. hypercalcemia
   d. hypocalcemia

99. Which of the following is **not** an early symptom of hypovolemia related to volume depletion?
   a. thirst
   b. muscle cramps
   c. postural dizziness
   d. salt craving

100. According to the American College of Surgeons surgical wound classification system, which of the following categories would a gunshot wound be classified as?
   a. class I
   b. class II
   c. class III
   d. class IV

101. Which of the following is an example of an enzymatic agent used in wound debridement?
   a. chlorhexidine
   b. collagenase
   c. becaplermin
   d. cadexomer iodine

102. Which of the following statements is **not** true regarding compartment syndrome?
   a. Pallor and pulselessness are early signs of compartment syndrome.
   b. Compartment syndrome can be either acute or chronic.
   c. Compartment syndrome most often occurs after a fracture, particularly a long bone fracture.
   d. The goal of treatment in compartment syndrome is decompression and the restoration of perfusion to the affected area.

103. Ventilator-associated pneumonia (VAP) is a healthcare associated infection that develops in a patient with an endotracheal tube or tracheostomy that has been mechanically ventilated for at least ___ hours when the infection is identified.
   a. 24 hours
   b. 72 hours
   c. 96 hours
   d. 48 hours

104. Which of the following best describes a minimally conscious state in patients who have experienced hypoxic-ischemic brain injury?
   a. no evidence of awareness of self or environment and an inability to interact with others
   b. no respiratory drive or spontaneous breathing
   c. patient is awake or aware but cannot move or communicate due to paralysis of muscles
   d. a severe alteration in consciousness with intermittent demonstration of restricted purposeful behavior and following commands

105. What does the "D" in the ABCD prioritization model for assessment of a trauma patient stand for?
    a. Disability
    b. Decompress
    c. Defibrillation
    d. Diagnose

106. Which of the following descriptions accurately describes a stage 2 pressure ulcer?
    a. The skin is intact with no evidence of pressure changes (including temperature, sensation and consistency).
    b. There is full thickness skin loss extending into the subcutaneous tissue.
    c. The wound is superficial with partial thickness skin loss involving the epidermis or dermis.
    d. There is extensive destruction including damage to muscle, bone, or supporting structures.

107. The majority of carbapenem-resistant *Enterobacteriaceae* (CRE) infections are caused by which organism?
    a. group A *Streptococcus*
    b. *Enterococcus faecium*
    c. *Aeromonas hydrophila*
    d. *Klebsiella pneumoniae*

108. Which of the following could be utilized as a preventative strategy in the management of cancer-related pain?
    a. Instruct the patient to only take prescribed analgesics when their pain level is moderate to severe to prevent narcotic dependency.
    b. The use of bone-modifying agents to prevent skeletal events including fractures and bone pain caused by bone metastases.
    c. Avoid the use of adjuvant agents or co-analgesics.
    d. The pharmacologic management of pain should begin with mild opioids.

109. Which of the following measures should be taken prior to the utilization of palliative sedation for a patient with terminal agitation?
    a. evaluation of the patient by the palliative care team
    b. pharmacologic management of agitation
    c. evaluation of patient by a psychiatrist
    d. all of the above

110. Allodynia is a characteristic used to describe pain. Which of the following best describes allodynia?
    a. A patient that states it is painful to brush her hair.
    b. A patient describes feeling as if her scalp is "on fire."
    c. A patient describes severe generalized pain "everywhere" after opioid discontinuation.
    d. A patient that is experiencing prolonged pain.

111. Which of the following treatments may be utilized to palliate respiratory distress in the dying patient?
   a. morphine sulfate
   b. administration of oxygen
   c. atropine
   d. all of the above

112. Which of the following best describes the principle of double effect?
   a. the correlated action of 2 or more medications
   b. the enhancement of the effect of a drug, treatment, or biologic
   c. the intentional painless ending of life of a patient suffering from an incurable and painful disease
   d. the administration of medication to relieve pain even if the unintended consequence is hastening of death by respiratory depression

113. Which of the following agents is **not** considered a vesicant?
   a. vancomycin
   b. methotrexate
   c. dobutamine
   d. propofol

114. Which of the following is **not** a potential cause of conductive hearing loss?
   a. auditory nerve damage
   b. lack of movement of small bones of inner ear
   c. fluid in the middle ear
   d. cerumen impaction

115. Which of the following hearing tests might be utilized to distinguish conductive hearing loss from sensorineural hearing loss?
   a. pneumoscopy
   b. CT scan of the temporal bone
   c. Weber and Rinne test
   d. audiogram

116. Which of the following outcomes is **not** associated with a NICHE program?
   a. decreased falls
   b. increased length of stay
   c. decreased restraint use
   d. decreased costs

117. Which of the following laboratory values is associated with salicylate toxicity?
   a. serum salicylate 10 mg/dL
   b. serum salicylate 20 mg/dL
   c. serum salicylate 30 mg/dL
   d. serum salicylate 45 mg/dL

118. You are rounding on a 62-year-old patient who arrived in the emergency department with abdominal pain, joint pain, and headache. His wife states that he has been exceptionally exhausted and irritable. The patient states that he is also experiencing some numbness and tingling in his toes. During the completion of the patient's health history, you learn that he is employed at a manufacturing plant that makes batteries. Which of the following laboratory tests might you order to help determine the cause of the patient's symptoms?
    a. toxicology screen
    b. blood alcohol level
    c. serum creatinine
    d. serum lead level

119. Which of the following criteria in patients with sepsis is indicative of septic shock?
    a. temperature > 38.3 degrees Celsius
    b. lactate > 2 mmol/L after adequate fluid resuscitation
    c. white blood cell count > 12,000
    d. tachypnea (> 20 respirations/minute)

120. Which of the following criteria is **not** part of the SOFA scale (sequential organ failure assessment) used to predict ICU mortality?
    a. platelet count
    b. Glasgow coma scale
    c. serum bilirubin
    d. lactic acid

121. Which of the following is **not** part of the criteria for the diagnosis of systemic inflammatory response syndrome (SIRS)?
    a. mean respiratory rate more than 2 standard deviations above normal for age
    b. tachycardia (defined as mean heart rate more than 2 standard deviations above normal for age)
    c. leukocyte count elevated or depressed for age
    d. core temperature of > 38 degrees Celsius

122. You are caring for a patient with chronic pain related to diabetic peripheral neuropathy. Which of the following classifications of medications might you consider prescribing to manage this type of pain?
    a. benzodiazepines
    b. antispasmodics
    c. tricyclic antidepressants
    d. serotonin-norepinephrine reuptake inhibitors

123. You are rounding on a 85-year-old patient at an extended care facility. She has a history of dementia and has recently been complaining of pain related to osteoarthritis. The patient's family is expressing concern that her mobility has been impacted by the pain. They are also concerned about the patient taking pain medication and have informed you that she is opioid-naïve. Which of the following would be an appropriate response to the patient's family regarding treatment of the patient's pain?
    a. "Given your mother's history of dementia, it is impossible to know if she is truly experiencing pain."
    b. "I am going to prescribe some immediate-release oxycodone for your mother's pain. She can have the medication every 4 to 6 hours as needed for pain."
    c. "I would like to start your mother on some scheduled acetaminophen for her osteoarthritis pain. We will see if this is effective over the next couple of days and if not we can make some modifications to her pain management regimen."
    d. "I suggest that we start your mother on some glucosamine and chondroitin for her. Due to her age and history of dementia, narcotics and nonsteroidal anti-inflammatory agents are contraindicated for pain management."

124. You are rounding on a 78-year-old male patient with dementia who is experiencing agitation and aggression. Which of the following pharmacological agents would be appropriate to order for the management of his agitation/aggression?
    a. diazepam
    b. rivastigmine
    c. diphenhydramine
    d. lorazepam

125. Which of the following is **not** a recommended strategy to mitigate the risk of delirium in the hospitalized patient?
    a. avoidance of medications that may precipitate delirium
    b. facilitation of sleep
    c. minimize cognitive stimulation
    d. orientation of patient

126. Which of the following is **not** considered to be a component of failure to thrive in elderly patients?
    a. disability
    b. dehydration
    c. impaired neuropsychiatric function
    d. physical frailty

127. The FRAIL scale is a mnemonic that can be utilized to assess frailty in an elderly patient. What does the "L" in the FRAIL scale represent?
    a. loss of weight
    b. loss of appetite
    c. low urine output
    d. leg pain

128. Which of the following statements is **not** true regarding elder mistreatment and abuse?
    a. The abuser is usually a family member (90% of the time).
    b. Elder mistreatment may involve the administration of inappropriate medications or incorrect dosages of medications.
    c. The highest rates of elder abuse are in women.
    d. Malnutrition, dehydration, and pressure ulcers may be warning signs of elder abuse.

129. The recommended treatment for obsessive-compulsive disorder is cognitive-behavioral therapy and which class of medication?
    a. selective serotonin reuptake inhibitor (SSRI)
    b. antipsychotic
    c. tricyclic antidepressant
    d. benzodiazepine

130. You are rounding on a 76-year-old male patient who was recently diagnosed with wet age-related macular degeneration (AMD) after experiencing significant visual changes. Which of the following treatment options would be appropriate for the treatment of wet AMD?
    a. topical prostaglandins
    b. topical beta-blockers
    c. intraocular lens implantation
    d. intravitreal bevacizumab

131. You are working in a heart failure clinic and frequently see Mr. Jones, a 79-year-old widower who has been coming to the clinic routinely for the past 6 months. Mr. Jones is often noncompliant with his medications and lifestyle modifications to control his heart failure symptoms. Which of the following strategies would **not** be appropriate to address Mr. Jones' nonadherence?
    a. Review the side effects of Mr. Jones' medications with him to see if they may be contributing to his nonadherence.
    b. Assess Mr. Jones' ability to pay for his medications.
    c. Provide Mr. Jones with education on his medications and lifestyle modifications and how they have improved his symptoms.
    d. Notify Mr. Jones' family that he is not competent to care for himself or make healthcare decisions because of his nonadherence.

132. Which of the following patient populations has the highest suicide rate in the United States?
    a. middle-aged white women 40 years and older
    b. young African-American men 25 years and older
    c. elderly white men 85 years and older
    d. Hispanic male adolescents 13 to 18 years old

133. Which of the following statements is **not** true regarding suicide screening in adult patients?
    a. Patients should not be questioned about suicidal thoughts by clinicians as this may prompt the patient to experience suicidal thoughts or actions.
    b. Psychiatric disorders, previous suicide attempts, and feelings of hopelessness are major risk factors for suicide.
    c. Social and family support help to decrease the risk of suicide.
    d. The first step in evaluating suicide risk is to determine the presence of suicidal thoughts.

134. The 5-step algorithm known as the five A's is often used to counsel patients in smoking cessation. Which of the following accurately describes the 5 A's?
   a. Advise, Assess, Adapt, Assist, Adopt
   b. Ask, Assess, Abate, Adapt, Assist
   c. Ask, Advise, Assess, Assist, Arrange
   d. Advise, Adjust, Assess, Arrange, Adopt

135. You are seeing a patient in the office who has expressed an interest in quitting smoking. He tells you that he has not pursued trying to quit in the past due to "not wanting to take any drugs to help me quit." Which of the following nonpharmacologic treatment options could you suggest to assist the patient in smoking cessation?
   a. behavioral counseling
   b. acupuncture
   c. hypnosis
   d. all of the above

136. All of the following are notable risk factors for obstructive sleep apnea except _____?
   a. advanced age
   b. female gender
   c. obesity
   d. craniofacial abnormality

137. You are a CNS working in an outpatient clinic and you are about to provide a patient with education on colon cancer screening. Which of the following statements by the patient indicates a need for further education regarding colon cancer screening recommendations?
   a. "I should begin getting screened at age 50."
   b. "My physician may order a colonoscopy or a test that detects blood in my stool as part of the screening process."
   c. "Since my brother has colorectal polyps, my physician may want to screen me sooner than age 50."
   d. "I will have a colonoscopy every 3 years as part of my screening for colon cancer."

138. Which of the following is true regarding a delayed hemolytic blood transfusion reaction?
   a. often occurs in patients who are receiving a blood product for the first time
   b. patients usually experience fever, chills, chest pain, and lower back pain during the transfusion
   c. transfused blood cells are broken down and destroyed days or weeks after the transfusion
   d. the patient's red blood cell count markedly increases after the transfusion

139. Which of the following considerations are relevant with the use of mannitol to reduce intracranial pressure and cerebral edema?
   a. Mannitol is a vesicant and care must be taken to avoid extravasation.
   b. Mannitol must be administered using a filter.
   c. Mannitol should be rapidly infused via a large peripheral vein.
   d. Mannitol is contraindicated for patients with severe heart failure
   e. a, b, and d

140. Certain viruses and bacteria have been linked in the development of various cancers. Which of the following is not a true statement regarding the link between viral infection and cancer development?
   a. *Helicobacter pylori* has been shown to increase the risk of gastric cancer.
   b. Hepatitis B and C increase the risk for liver cancer.
   c. Human papillomavirus (HPV) increases the risk for cervical cancer.
   d. Cytomegalovirus increases the risk of renal cell carcinoma.

141. Which of the following best describes "culturally competent" care?
   a. the clinical skills/professional behaviors of a clinician that focus on the cultural beliefs, values, and perceptions of the patient during the therapeutic relationship established between the patient and clinician
   b. a way of life belonging to an individual or group of individuals that reflects values and customs
   c. recognition that each individual is unique along the dimensions of race, gender, ethnicity, religious beliefs, and sexual orientation
   d. the adoption of the elements of one culture by members of a different culture

142. You are rounding on an intensive care step-down unit and one of the registered nurses approaches you visibly upset. She states that she is caring for a 42-year-old female patient with a dangerously low hemoglobin level. The patient is a Jehovah's Witness and is refusing blood products. The RN shares with you that she had a discussion with the patient this afternoon that has upset the patient. She states that she told the patient she must reconsider receiving a blood transfusion or she may not survive. She states that she told the patient that other patients receive blood products routinely and it is very safe. Which of the following terms best describes the interaction between the RN and the patient?
   a. cultural blindness
   b. cultural competence
   c. cultural imposition
   d. ethnocentrism

143. Cultural imposition or lack of sensitivity may lead to which of the following?
   a. acculturation
   b. cultural pain
   c. culture shock
   d. cultural blindness

144. An example of a professional behavior of a culturally competent practitioner would be:
   a. recognition of the daily religious practices of a Muslim patient
   b. recognition of the dietary needs of a Jewish patient
   c. recognition of the prominence of cardiovascular disease among African Americans
   d. all of the above

145. You are working in a large inner city medical center where patients with a low health literacy level are common. Which of the following strategies could you implement in formatting new patient education materials?
   a. print materials at an 8th grade reading level
   b. print educational material with graphics only
   c. print educational materials in bright colors and a larger font
   d. utilize short, simple sentences and summarize key points at the end of a section

146. You are caring for a 92-year-old patient who was admitted to the orthopedic unit after a fall at home with a fracture. Ensuring the patient's pain is immediately addressed and appropriately managed is an example of which ethical principle?
   a. nonmaleficence
   b. justice
   c. beneficence
   d. autonomy

147. You are working in a skilled nursing facility and observe one of the registered nurses administering medications to Mrs. J, one of the residents. Mrs. J. is a 72-year-old patient currently residing at the facility after suffering a stroke and requiring rehabilitation. She is alert and oriented to person, place, and time, and competent to make decisions. You overhear Mrs. J. tell the registered nurse that she does not want to take her Colace today since she had a loose bowel movement this morning. The registered nurse tells the patient, "Your doctor wants you to have this medication so you need to take it." Which ethical principle is this nurse violating?
   a. nonmaleficence
   b. justice
   c. beneficence
   d. autonomy

148. Which of the following legislative actions was designed to ensure that patients are informed of their rights to accept or refuse medical care and execute advanced directives?
   a. Health Insurance Portability and Accountability Act
   b. Patient Self-Determination Act
   c. Oregon's Death with Dignity Act
   d. Genetic Information Nondiscrimination Act

149. Which of the following actions could constitute a violation of patient rights?
   a. failing to provide a limited English proficiency patient with an interpreter
   b. failing to manage a patient's pain
   c. failing to provide a patient with information regarding their treatment plan
   d. all of the above

150. You are caring for an 83-year-old male patient with advanced cancer. The patient has expressed wanting to die at home, despite objections from his son who wants him to remain hospitalized. Which of the following interventions would be appropriate to advocate for this patient and his wishes?
   a. Explain to the patient that his son has power of attorney and he needs to remain in the hospital.
   b. Arrange a family meeting with the patient and his son along with the palliative care team to discuss his plan of care.
   c. Discharge the patient to an inpatient hospice care center.
   d. Consult the hospital ethics committee.

151. Which of the following critical thinking skills is associated with the assessment piece of the nursing process?
    a. differentiate between relevant and irrelevant data
    b. organize and categorize data into patterns or groups
    c. determine the patient's level of progress
    d. revise the plan of care

152. Which of the following best describes systems thinking?
    a. the analysis and evaluation of information, beliefs, and knowledge
    b. focusing on a limited number of choices or possibilities
    c. the breaking down of a complex problem into single components
    d. an analysis of the relationships between a system's parts in an effort to view the system holistically and explain its behavior

153. The use of systems thinking by nursing in health care has the potential to impact which of the following?
    a. mitigate errors
    b. enhance quality improvement initiatives
    c. improve delegation
    d. all of the above

154. You are providing education to the nursing staff regarding systems thinking. Which of the following statements by one of your students indicates a need for further clarification?
    a. "Systems thinking cannot be measured."
    b. "Systems thinking is often utilized in quality improvement initiatives."
    c. "Systems thinking links a person's environment to his/her behavior."
    d. "Problems occur as part of a chain of events in a larger system."

155. Which of the following approaches/strategies might be utilized to teach nursing staff about systems thinking?
    a. participation in a root cause analysis
    b. review of case studies
    c. creating a flowchart
    d. all of the above

156. You are working to develop, plan, and implement an educational program on nutrition for geriatric patients. Using Malcolm Knowles' theory of adult learning to guide the process, which of the following statement is applicable to the development of your program?
    a. The program will include activities that encourage active participation of the participants.
    b. The program will include an outline of the goals and objectives of the course.
    c. The program will include a discussion at the beginning of the course allowing the participants to share past experiences in how they have utilized healthy eating habits.
    d. all of the above

157. Which of the following strategies should be utilized for teaching geriatric adults in a group setting?
   a. Do not wait until the end of the presentation to address questions. Answer questions throughout the presentation.
   b. Use the teach back technique to confirm understanding.
   c. Avoid frequent breaks to minimize distractions.
   d. Avoid the use of handouts.

158. Which of the following physical or physiologic changes has the potential to affect an older adult's learning?
   a. stress
   b. fatigue
   c. limited mobility or range of motion
   d. all of the above

159. Which of the following best describes the definition of the term androgogy?
   a. a theory of group of ideas about how something should be done
   b. an individual's ability to read and write
   c. the process of stimulating and helping older people learn
   d. the unique characteristics of teaching and learning of adults

160. You are preparing to provide patient education to a newly diagnosed type 2 diabetic Hispanic patient who has limited English proficiency. Which of the following strategies might you utilize to ensure the teaching is effective for this patient?
   a. written materials in both English and Spanish
   b. including family in teaching sessions
   c. one-on-one education session
   d. all of the above

161. In the Iowa Model of Evidence-Based Practice to Promote Quality Care, the perspective of the steps in the evidence-based practice process is from the viewpoint of the _____.
   a. patient
   b. clinician
   c. researcher
   d. administrator

162. Which of the following definitions best describes translation science?
   a. a set of concepts, definitions, relationships and propositions derived from nursing models or other disciplines that project a purposive systematic view of phenomena
   b. the integration of best research evidence, clinical expertise, and patient values to guide clinical care
   c. a theory or group of ideas about how something should be done or thought about
   d. the investigation of methods, variables, and interventions that influence the adoption of evidence-based practices to improve clinical and operational decision making

163. In nurse theorist Katharine Kolcaba's theory of comfort, she describes comfort existing in 3 forms. They include:
    a. repose, ease, contentment
    b. solace, contentment, relief
    c. relaxation, repose, tranquility
    d. relief, ease and transcendence

164. You are working with a fellow clinical nurse specialist on the geriatric unit. The nurse manager approaches you both and requests that you assist her this afternoon with providing some staff education at the scheduled staff meeting. Your colleague is visibly frustrated and tells the nurse manager that today is not really a good day for her, given her busy schedule. The nurse manager does not acknowledge your colleague's comments and states, "Well I appreciate your flexibility," and walks away. Which of the following conflict management strategies did the nurse manager utilize?
    a. dominating
    b. avoiding
    c. obliging
    d. compromising

165. You are having an issue with one of your CNS colleagues regarding how patients are divided and assigned to the clinical nurse specialists on the unit. Which of the following statements would be most appropriate to utilize when addressing this issue with your colleague?
    a. "You never divide the assignment fairly."
    b. "I really like working with you but I feel the workload is not being fairly divided."
    c. "I really enjoy working here and with you. I am hoping we can take a look at the way we complete the assignment to make the workload manageable for the both of us."
    d. "I have noticed that you always have the fewest number of patients in your assignment. Can we please discuss?"

166. Which of the following is a recommended communication strategy that can be utilized in conflict resolution?
    a. use of closed-ended questions
    b. being subjective
    c. including the individual in the definition of the problem
    d. speaking low and slowly, using relaxed body language

167. Which of the following principles does **not** define patient-centered care?
    a. viewing the patient as a whole person
    b. patient satisfaction
    c. addressing a patient's need for information
    d. consideration of a patient's ability to understand

168. Which of the following skill sets useful in providing patient-centered care is defined as "the ability of a person to recognize, understand, and evaluate their own emotions, as well as the emotions of others to guide their thinking and actions"?
    a. cultural competence
    b. interpersonal communication
    c. emotional intelligence
    d. cultural sensitivity

169. There are 3 pillars defined in the World Health Organization's falls prevention model. Which of the following is **not** a pillar of the model?
    a. building awareness
    b. encouraging behavioral changes
    c. identifying and assessing risk
    d. identifying and implementing realistic and effective interventions

170. Which of the following is **not** a risk factor in the development of osteoporosis?
    a. late menopause
    b. low calcium intake
    c. smoking
    d. white race

171. You are providing education to a group of registered nurses on evidence-based practice. Which of the following barriers to adopting evidence-based practice might you encounter from the staff?
    a. lack of time
    b. inability to understand statistical terminology
    c. inadequate understanding of research
    d. all of the above

172. Which of the following is not one of the 5 competencies that the Institute of Medicine recommended in their 2011 report, *The Future of Nursing: Leading Change, Advancing Health*, for all healthcare professionals to possess?
    a. patient-centered care
    b. evidence-based practice
    c. quality improvement
    d. nursing theory

173. Which of the following is **not** a key component of evidence-based practice?
    a. clinical expertise
    b. personal experience
    c. research evidence
    d. patient values

174. You are practicing as a geriatric clinical nurse specialist in a large academic medication center. You have noticed recently that there has been an increase in the number of falls on your unit in the last 3 months. You would like to review the types of fall intervention strategies in the literature to see what interventions might be effective. Now that you have begun the inquiry process, what is the next step in the evidence-based practice process?
    a. search for the best evidence
    b. evaluate outcomes
    c. ask clinical questions using patient scenarios
    d. integrate the clinical evidence into practice

175. Which of the following physiologic conditions might affect the distribution of medications across body compartments in an elderly patient?
    a. decreased fat mass
    b. increased muscle mass
    c. decreased body water
    d. increased serum albumin

# Answers and Explanations

1. **D:** Headache, disorientation, confusion, and epistaxis are all symptoms that may be associated with hypertension. The incidence of hypertension increases with advancing age and may occur in up to 60% to 80% of patients age 60 years and older. Hypertension is typically defined as a systolic pressure > 140 mm Hg and a diastolic pressure > 90 mm Hg. Male gender is a risk factor for hypertension.

2. **A:** Patients experiencing a hypertensive crisis should have their blood pressure decreased over a period of hours to days. Elderly patients may require even slower reductions to decrease the risk of cerebral and myocardial ischemia. In hypertensive patients who have not been previously treated for hypertension, antihypertensive therapy should be initiated and may consist of a calcium channel blocker, beta-blocker, angiotensin-converting enzyme (ACE) inhibitor, angiotensin II receptor blocker (ARB), or a combination of these agents. Sublingual nifedipine is contraindicated in patients with hypertensive crisis. Nonpharmacologic treatment options such as rest and a quiet environment may help to decrease blood pressure.

3. **C:** Elevated levels of HDL cholesterol lower the risk of cardiovascular disease. A level greater than or equal to 60 mg/dL is desirable, while HDL levels less than 40 mg/dL may increase the risk of cardiovascular disease. Reducing foods that contain a high level of cholesterol such as eggs and organ meats is recommended. HMG-CoA reductase inhibitors, also known as "statins," may cause myopathies that manifest as muscle pain and weakness and patients should be taught to report these symptoms to their healthcare provider. Grapefruit and grapefruit juice should be limited in patients taking a HMG-CoA reductase inhibitor, as they may increase the risk of side effects of the medication.

4. **B:** Cardiac tamponade. Cardiac tamponade occurs when blood or fluid fills the pericardium, putting excess pressure on the myocardium and preventing the ventricles from fully expanding. As a result, the heart does not effectively pump, decreasing perfusion. Risk factors for cardiac tamponade include myocardial infarction, malignancy, dissecting aortic aneurysm, cardiac surgery or invasive cardiac procedures, pericarditis, renal failure, or cardiac trauma. Patients experiencing cardiac tamponade will have symptoms of hypoperfusion including hypotension, tachycardia, tachypnea, and elevated jugular venous pressure. In addition, patients may experience weak or absent pulses, cool, clammy skin, drowsiness, and dyspnea.

5. **D:** Acute coronary syndrome (ACS) is a clinical presentation that includes both unstable angina as well as ST-elevation and non-ST-elevation myocardial infarctions (MI). According to the American Heart Association guidelines on the Acute Coronary Care in the Elderly, age is a strong predictor of outcome with the odds for an in-hospital death for an ACS patient increasing by 70% for every 10 years of age. Elderly ACS patients are less likely to receive evidence-based interventions, and medical advances in the treatment of ACS have primarily been recognized in younger people (< 65 years of age).

6. **C:** Administration of morphine sulfate. Acute decompensated heart failure occurs when the body cannot compensate for the heart's inability to provide adequate perfusion. Cardiac output is no longer sufficient to meet the metabolic demands of the body. Acute heart failure occurs suddenly and can be precipitated by dysrhythmias, illness, noncompliance with medications, acute ischemia, fluid overload, or hypertensive crisis. It requires immediate treatment to restore adequate perfusion and is often life-threatening. Treatment options include the administration of diuretics and vasodilators, airway assessment with continuous pulse oximetry, supplemental oxygen and

potential ventilatory support, sodium restriction, urine output monitoring, and continuous cardiac monitoring. Opiate therapy is not recommended for patients with acute decompensated heart failure.

7. A: systemic vascular resistance is decreased. The myocardium of older adults becomes stiff and more rigid with age, thereby compromising cardiac output. This also results in increased afterload on the left ventricle, an increase in systolic blood pressure, and left ventricular hypertrophy. The myocardium is also less sensitive to catecholamines in the older adult. Systemic vascular resistance is increased and often contributes to baseline hypertension.

8. B: *Staphylococcus aureus*. Older adults with endocarditis are more likely to experience a poorer prognosis. Although gram-negative organisms such as *Escherichia coli*, *Proteus* species, and *Klebsiella* species are some of the most common organisms causing endocarditis, *Staphylococcus aureus* is the most common gram-positive organism and is associated with the highest mortality rate.

9. B: Cardiogenic shock is more common in non-ST elevation MI patients. Cardiogenic shock is the most common cause of death in patients with acute myocardial infarctions, with ST-elevation MI patients having a greater risk of cardiogenic shock than non-ST-elevation MI patients. MI with failure of the left ventricle is the most common cause of cardiogenic shock. Hypoperfusion is the hallmark sign of cardiogenic shocks and symptoms may include decreased urinary output and mental status change. Pulmonary artery catheterization is often used to diagnose cardiogenic shock.

10. E: All of the above. Cardiogenic pulmonary edema occurs when an accumulation of fluid enters the interstitium of the lung and alveoli related to cardiac dysfunction. Left ventricular systolic dysfunction is a common cause of cardiogenic pulmonary edema. Left ventricular diastolic dysfunction and dysrhythmias, such as new-onset rapid atrial fibrillation and ventricular tachycardia, may also cause cardiogenic pulmonary edema. Mechanical complications from myocardial infarctions may contribute to the development of cardiogenic pulmonary edema as well.

11. E: All of the above. Inflammatory conditions are associated with atrial fibrillation and there is a positive correlation between C-reactive protein and atrial fibrillation. Hyperthyroidism increases the risk of atrial fibrillation, although the exact mechanism is unknown. Chronic kidney disease and atrial fibrillation often occur together and chronic kidney disease patients with atrial fibrillation are more likely to progress to renal failure than those without atrial fibrillation. Hiatal hernias may compress the left atrium, contributing to the development of atrial fibrillation. In addition, hiatal hernias are often associated with gastroesophageal reflux, which is also potentially a trigger for the development of atrial fibrillation.

12. C: Poorly controlled hypertension. Patients with asymptomatic carotid artery stenosis who have the following characteristics may be at an increased risk of stroke: male gender, current smoking, poorly controlled hypertension, or history of contralateral transient ischemic attack or stroke.

13. D: Peripheral neuropathy. Acute peripheral arterial insufficiency can occur as a result of traumatic injury (including crushing injuries) and nontraumatic events such as arterial thrombus or embolism. When sudden occlusion of the vessel occurs, tissue ischemia develops, which can ultimately lead to cellular death. Ischemia is caused by a reduction of oxygenation to the tissue as a result of compromised blood flow. Compromised blood flow prevents the transport of essential nutrients to the cells. Risk factors for acute peripheral arterial insufficiency include age, tobacco use, diabetes mellitus, hyperlipidemia, and hypertension. Signs and symptoms of acute arterial

insufficiency include the 6 P's: pain (often extreme), pallor, pulselessness, poikilothermic (the inability to regulate body temperature), paresthesia, and paralysis. Paresthesia and paralysis are usually late signs of arterial insufficiency.

14. B: Restrictive cardiomyopathy. Restrictive cardiomyopathy occurs when the ventricles do not relax and the filling of the ventricles is restricted. This type of cardiomyopathy causes the ventricles to become stiff and rigid and impede ventricular function. Wall thickness is not affected. Hypertrophic cardiomyopathy occurs when the cardiac muscle enlarges and thickens, making the heart unable to pump blood effectively. Dilated cardiomyopathy occurs when the ventricles become enlarged and weaken. The term idiopathic cardiomyopathy may be used when the cause of the cardiomyopathy cannot be determined.

15. A: Ebstein's anomaly. Ebstein's anomaly involves the malformation of the tricuspid valve, which causes blood to leak back into the right atrium. Mild forms of Ebstein's anomaly may not cause symptoms until later in adulthood. Symptoms are often likely to develop slowly over many years. An atrial septal defect occurs when part of the atrial septum does not form properly, leaving a hole in the septum. Patent ductus arteriosus occurs when the temporary blood vessel formed in utero known as the ductus arteriosus remains open after birth. The ductus arteriosus normally seals off after birth to prevent the mixing of blood from the aorta and pulmonary artery. Coarctation of the aorta is a narrowing of the aorta that restricts blood flow through the aorta, resulting in hypertension.

16. A: Aortic dissection. Aortic dissection is a complication that can occur postoperatively after a coronary artery bypass graft. Patients who are elderly, have longstanding hypertension, severely narrowed coronary arteries, or widening of the aorta are at greater risk. Pleural effusions are common after a coronary artery bypass graft and rarely require treatment. Phrenic nerve damage is a rare complication causing diaphragmatic dysfunction and/or paralysis. Thrombocytopenia may occur from the heparin administered before, during, and after the procedure.

17. C: Coronary artery injuries are the most common type of blunt cardiac injury. Blunt cardiac injuries are most commonly seen in trauma situations whereby a patient experiences a significant force to the chest, causing damage to the heart itself. Blunt cardiac injuries are often associated with other thoracic injuries and the majority of patients are asymptomatic after the injury occurs. More severe blunt cardiac injuries may lead to exsanguination, pericardial tamponade, and death. The most common type of blunt cardiac injury is a myocardial contusion.

18. C: Increased fibrinolysis. In elderly patients, certain physiologic changes have the potential to increase the risk of bleeding associated with antithrombotic therapy. Increased clotting, decreased fibrinolysis, and polypharmacy resulting in drug-drug interactions are all factors that may increase the patient's risk of bleeding on antithrombotic therapy. In addition, renal function decreases with age and therefore may contribute to an accumulation of certain antithrombotic agents, increasing the risk of bleeding.

19. D: Pneumothorax should be suspected in any patient with penetrating chest trauma. Blunt chest trauma is generally more common than penetrating chest trauma; however, penetrating chest trauma is more deadly. Penetrating chest trauma most often occurs from gunshots and stabbings. Most penetrating chest injuries do not require major surgical intervention. Pneumothorax is an important consideration in all patients with penetrating chest trauma. A small pneumothorax may be difficult to detect clinically.

20. A: Healthcare professionals should consider discontinuing medications containing saxagliptin and alogliptin in patients who develop heart failure, and should monitor their diabetes control. The FDA MedWatch alert for patients taking dipeptidyl peptidase-4 inhibitors that contain saxagliptin and alogliptin recommends that healthcare professionals should consider discontinuing medications containing saxagliptin and alogliptin in patients who develop heart failure and should monitor their diabetes control. Patients experiencing shortness of breath, fatigue, weight gain, and swelling should contact their healthcare professional right away. They should not stop taking their medication without consulting with their healthcare professional. Dipeptidyl peptidase 4-inhibitors are used with diet and exercise to lower blood glucose in adults with type 2 diabetes.

21. C: Saddle. A saddle pulmonary embolism lodges at the bifurcation of the main pulmonary artery and extends into the left and right pulmonary arteries. Segmental and subsegmental pulmonary emboli occur in the segmental and subsegmental pulmonary arteries. Hemodynamically stable pulmonary emboli are defined as a pulmonary embolism that does not present with hypotension, hypotension requiring vasopressors, or clear evidence of shock.

22. B: Intravenous fluid resuscitation. This patient meets the criteria for hemodynamically unstable pulmonary embolism (hypotension (SBP < 90 mm Hg) for a period of > 15 minutes, hypotension requiring vasopressors, or clear evidence of shock). The initial support for the hemodynamically unstable patient is the restoration of tissue perfusion with intravenous fluid resuscitation, vasopressor support (when fluid resuscitation is ineffective), and oxygenation. Placement of an inferior vena cava filter is not a necessary treatment option for most patients. Embolectomy may be an appropriate treatment option for patients who fail thrombolytic therapy or who are not candidates.

23. D: All of the above. Cardiomegaly may be seen on chest x-ray in up to 50% of patients with a diagnosis of pulmonary embolism. Atelectasis is another common finding, with up to 69% of patients with a pulmonary embolism showing atelectasis on chest x-ray. Up to 22% of patients with pulmonary embolism will have a normal chest x-ray.

24. B: Pulmonary function tests. Chest x-ray, pulmonary function tests, electrocardiography, and a complete blood cell count may be used to confirm a diagnosis of asthma in the older adult patient. Pulmonary function tests are the most useful diagnostic test in confirming a diagnosis of asthma and differentiating between other respiratory diagnoses such as chronic obstructive pulmonary disease. Chest x-ray usually results in negative findings for the asthmatic patient; however, other abnormalities may be detected. Electrocardiography may be utilized to determine the presence of underlying cardiac disease and assist the healthcare practitioner with ordering the appropriate medication if a diagnosis of asthma is made. Computed tomography (CT) scanning may be useful for patients with recurring symptoms or chronic disease.

25. A: Losartan. Angiotensin-converting enzyme (ACE) inhibitors may exacerbate asthma symptoms, most commonly producing cough. Monoamine oxidase inhibitors and tricyclic antidepressants used in the treatment of depression have the potential to interact with corticosteroids and worsen depression. Angiotensin II receptor blockers do not have the same effect as ACE inhibitors on asthma symptoms and are the preferred treatment option along with calcium channel blockers for asthmatic patients with hypertension. Pantoprazole does not produce or contribute to the exacerbation of asthma symptoms.

26. D: Thyroid disease. There are multiple diseases and conditions that can cause dyspnea to occur, including cardiac and pulmonary diseases, anemia, thyroid disease, and psychogenic causes.

Palpitations, generalized fatigue, and heat intolerance are symptoms that are indicative of thyrotoxicosis. Pallor, fatigue, and evidence of blood loss indicate anemia. Chest pain, syncope, and fatigue may indicate aortic stenosis. Psychogenic dyspnea usually occurs at rest and may be accompanied by peripheral and periorbital paresthesias.

27. C: Patients with idiopathic arterial hypertension. WHO group 1 patients are defined as patients with idiopathic arterial hypertension. Group 2 patients are defined as patients with pulmonary hypertension secondary to left-sided heart disease. Group 3 patients are defined as patients with pulmonary hypertension secondary to hypoxemia or chronic lung disease. Patients with group 4 pulmonary hypertension have pulmonary hypertension secondary to thromboembolic occlusion of the pulmonary vasculature. Patients in group 5 have pulmonary hypertension due to unknown or unclear mechanisms.

28. B: Obesity. There are multiple risk factors that may increase the likelihood of developing obstructive sleep apnea. Obesity is the most common risk factor for obstructive sleep apnea in both males and females. Male gender, smoking, craniofacial and upper airway abnormalities, increasing age, and menopause are other risk factors. In addition, there are medical conditions that may also increase risk, including heart failure, hypothyroidism, and renal disease.

29. D: Moxifloxacin. Clindamycin is the drug of choice for first-line therapy in the treatment of aspiration pneumonia caused by anaerobic bacteria. Other alternate treatment options include Amoxicillin-clavulanate or metronidazole plus amoxicillin or penicillin G. Moxifloxacin may be an effective treatment; however, it is an agent that is not preferred as first-line therapy in the treatment of aspiration pneumonia caused by anaerobic bacteria.

30. A: Right main stem bronchus. Treatment of aspiration of foreign bodies is highly dependent on the size of the foreign body its location. The right main stem bronchus is the most common site of foreign body aspiration. Foreign bodies lodged in the oropharynx or trachea are likely to cause acute asphyxiation, depending on the size of the foreign body. Foreign bodies are more likely to be aspirated in the lower lobes, causing distal bronchial obstruction.

31. D: Marked airflow obstruction on spirometry. Indications for lung volume reduction surgery for patients with emphysema include (but are not limited to) age younger than 75 years, severe dyspnea that persists after medical therapy and maximal pulmonary rehabilitation, and marked airflow obstruction on spirometry. Inability to complete a 6- to 10-week pulmonary rehabilitation program is a contraindication for lung volume reduction surgery in patients with emphysema.

32. D: Treatment with glucocorticoids. Treatment-related predictors of mortality in acute respiratory distress syndrome include a positive fluid balance, late intubation, packed red blood cell transfusion, and glucocorticoid treatment prior to the development of acute respiratory distress syndrome. In addition, patients with acute respiratory distress syndrome admitted to intensive care units without mandated care by an intensivist has shown to increase mortality risk.

33. A: Interstitial pneumonia. Pulmonary interstitial emphysema (PIE) may occur in patients with acute respiratory distress syndrome or mechanically ventilated patients. PIE is characterized by the dissection of air through the alveolar walls into the interstitial tissues, causing inflammation. Pulmonary interstitial emphysema is most commonly seen in patients with usual interstitial pneumonia. There may also be a correlation with prior ventilation and/or lung biopsy and the development of PIE.

34. B: Observation. Research supports treating asymptomatic patients with occult pneumothorax less than 8 mm in length with observation alone. In the event that the patient becomes symptomatic or the pneumothorax enlarges, placement of a chest tube would be indicated. Positive-pressure ventilation may contribute to the expansion of the pneumothorax and should only be initiated in patients with traumatic pneumothorax with a chest tube in place.

35. D: Elevation of the hemidiaphragm. Anatomical changes for patients undergoing a pneumonectomy include elevation of the hemidiaphragm, shifting of the mediastinum towards the post-pneumonectomy and hyperinflation of the remaining lung. Rapid accumulation of fluid into the post-pneumonectomy space may indicate hemorrhage or infection. Obliteration of the post-pneumonectomy space rarely occurs with most patients having residual fluid or air within the space.

36. B: Secondary polycythemia. As compensation for the decreased amount of oxygen in chronic obstructive pulmonary disease, the body makes extra red blood cells. This is known as secondary polycythemia and results in an excess number of circulating red blood cells. The excess red blood cells thicken the blood and clog small blood vessels. This results in the development of cyanosis. Cor pulmonale occurs when the right ventricle enlarges and thickens. Mucus hypersecretion and tissue destruction in chronic obstructive pulmonary disease cause airway inflammation and fibrosis.

37. D: Bartter syndrome. There are several familial/congenital conditions that are associated with the development of central diabetes insipidus (CDI). They include familial central diabetes insipidus, Wolfram syndrome, congenital hypopituitarism, and septo-optic dysplasia. Bartter syndrome is a congenital condition that is associated with the development of nephrogenic diabetes insipidus.

38. A: Beta-blockers. ACE inhibitors, beta-blockers, quinolone antibiotics, and salicylates are all medications that have the potential to cause hypoglycemia. In addition, alcohol ingestion may also contribute to hypoglycemia. Estrogens, sympathomimetics, and phenothiazines are all associated with the development of hyperglycemia.

39. D: Infusion of isotonic saline. Infusion of isotonic saline is the recommended first step in the treatment of diabetic ketoacidosis and hyperglycemic hyperosmolar state, followed immediately by administration of potassium replacement (if serum potassium level is less than 5.3). Isotonic saline increases insulin responsiveness and expands cardiovascular volume. IV insulin analogues may be administered as an alternative to insulin in the treatment of diabetic ketoacidosis. IV insulin should not be initiated in patients with a potassium level less than 3.3 until the potassium has been replaced. Insulin has the potential to further lower serum potassium levels when administered in the hypokalemic patient. Administration of sodium bicarbonate may be indicated if the patient's arterial pH is low (less than 6.9).

40. D: Plasmapheresis. A diagnosis of thyroid storm may be life-threatening and requires multiple treatment strategies. Administration of a beta-blocker is used to control symptoms (including tachycardia and cardiac arrhythmias). Administration of an iodine solution will help to decrease thyroid hormone. Glucocorticoids reduce T4 to T3 conversion. Plasmapheresis is a treatment option for thyroid storm that may be used when traditional treatment options fail and is not usually seen as first-line therapy.

41. A: Treatment goal of hemoglobin A1c < 7% with metformin and lifestyle intervention is not achieved within 3 months. According to the American Diabetes Association and European

Association for the Study of Diabetes, the addition of a secondary medication is recommended when the treatment goal of hemoglobin A1c of 7% with metformin and lifestyle intervention is not achieved within 3 months. Factors such as comorbidities and life expectancy may prohibit a patient from reaching this goal, therefore the treatment goal of hemoglobin A1c < 7% may not be appropriate for all patients. Targeted glycemic goals may need to be adjusted in the older adult based on these factors.

42. C: Bromocriptine. Bromocriptine is a dopamine agonist traditionally used in the treatment of Parkinson disease. It is not a recommended treatment option for type 2 diabetes due to its frequent gastrointestinal side effects and overall ineffectiveness in lowering hemoglobin A1c. There are many other medications in the treatment of type 2 diabetes that have been proven more effective.

43. A: Patients with severe neurologic symptoms require a slow correction of hyponatremia. The treatment of SIADH involves both the treatment of the underlying disease as well as therapy to increase the serum sodium level. The treatment of SIADH is also determined by the severity of the symptoms. Patients with severe neurologic symptoms require a more rapid correction of hyponatremia than those with mild or moderate symptoms. Patients with mild neurologic symptoms may be treated with fluid restriction and oral salt tablets. Treatment of patients with asymptomatic hyponatremia should focus on the underlying cause and may only be treated with fluid restriction (if cause cannot be determined.) Fluid restriction is a hallmark therapy for SIADH with the goal fluid intake of less than 800 mL/day.

44. B: Knee. Septic arthritis is defined as an invasion of the joint space by bacteria, virus, or fungi. Elderly patients, immunosuppressed patients, and those with prosthetic joints are at increased risk of the development of septic arthritis. The most commonly affected joints include the knee (most common), hip, shoulder, ankle, and wrist. Signs and symptoms of septic arthritis include joint pain, fever, impaired range of motion, chills, edema, erythema, warmth, and the abnormal presence of fluid (effusion) surrounding the joint. Treatment for septic arthritis is the administration of antibiotics. Surgical irrigation and debridement may also be indicated. The patient with septic arthritis will likely undergo physical therapy as part of their recovery to improve and restore mobility and range of motion.

45. F: A and C. Rhabdomyolysis occurs when damage of the cells of the skeletal muscles causes the release of toxins from injured cells into the bloodstream. Rhabdomyolysis may be caused by trauma, tissue ischemia, infection, certain medications (such as statins used for the lowering of cholesterol, selective serotonin reuptake inhibitors, lithium, and antihistamines), sepsis, immobilization, extraordinary physical exertion, myopathies, and cocaine or alcohol abuse. Additionally, rhabdomyolysis may occur with exposure to certain toxins such as snake or insect venoms or mushroom poisoning. In rare circumstances, the identifiable cause cannot be determined. The most serious complication of rhabdomyolysis is renal failure.

46. C: Functional tremor. Functional movement disorders are defined as an involuntary, abnormal movement of part of the body in which pathophysiology is not fully understood. Functional tremors are the most frequent type of functional movement disorder. Functional tremors (also known as psychogenic tremors) are involuntary muscle movements caused by an underlying psychological condition. Dystonia, myoclonus, and parkinsonism are other types of functional movement disorders. Functional gait disorders are another type of functional movement disorder and are common in the elderly.

47. D: Cautious gait. Gait disorders can manifest as a dragging gait, knee buckling, small slow steps or "walking on ice," swaying gait, fluctuating gait, hesitant gait, and hyperkinetic gait in which there is excessive movement of the arms, trunk, and legs when ambulating. Patients with gait disorders are at an increased risk of falling. Gait disorders are diagnosed by a thorough clinical examination (including a neurologic assessment) and history. Cautious gait does not necessarily indicate a functional gait disorder, but rather a psychological response to fear of falling and/or changes in equilibrium.

48. B: Falls. Falls are the leading cause of death from injury in men and women older than 65 years. Death rates attributed to falls were the highest for both men and women, with the rates for men 1.4 times higher than the rates for women. Motor vehicle accidents, suffocation, poisoning, and fire were amongst the top 5 causes of death from unintentional injury.

49. A: Compartment syndrome. Compartment syndrome occurs when there is an increase in the amount of pressure within a grouping of muscles, nerves, and blood vessels, resulting in compromised blood flow to muscles and nerves. If left untreated, tissue ischemia and eventual tissue death will occur. Compartment syndrome most often occurs after a fracture, particularly a long bone fracture. Risk factors for the development of compartment syndrome also include lower extremity trauma, massive tissue injury, venous obstruction, the use of certain medications (anticoagulants), burns, and compressive dressings or casts. Compartment syndrome can also occur with crush syndrome and rhabdomyolysis.

50. D: The measurement of intracompartmental pressures. The diagnosis of compartment syndrome is made by physical assessment and the measurement of intracompartmental pressures. Although laboratory abnormalities may develop, laboratory findings are not used in the diagnosis of compartment syndrome. Radiologic testing may be conducted to rule out other causes of symptoms; however, this testing is not usually found to be useful in the diagnosis of compartment syndrome.

51. D: Hypercalcemia. Superior vena cava syndrome is characterized by edema of the face, neck, and upper extremities, respiratory compromise, chest pain, headache, dizziness, and feeling of facial fullness. The clinical features of septic shock include tachypnea, nausea, diarrhea, and confusion. As the septic shock progresses, oliguria and metabolic acidosis occur. Although the patient may experience some of the symptoms listed above with metastasis to the liver, hypercalcemia is the oncologic complication that presents with the clinical presentation of mental status change, weakness, nausea, vomiting, constipation, and abdominal pain. In addition, small cell lung cancer is a malignancy commonly associated with hypercalcemia.

52. B: The use of bone-modifying agents to prevent skeletal events including fractures and bone pain caused by bone metastases. The use of bone-modifying agents are considered standard treatment in patients with lytic bone lesions. The use of these agents can prevent skeletal fractures and bone pain caused by metastasis. Bisphosphonates inhibit osteoclast-mediated bone resorption. Patients should be educated on taking analgesics around the clock to prevent pain. According to the World Health Organization 3-step analgesic ladder, adjuvant agents should be used to treat symptoms associated with pain such as anxiety or depression. Pharmacologic management of pain should begin with nonopioid therapy and progress to the use of opioids when pain persists or increases.

53. C: 80 fL. Mean corpuscular volume (MCV) is the measurement of the average size of a red blood cell. The normal range of mean corpuscular volume is 80 to 100 femtoliters. MCV less than 80 fL is

indicative of smaller than normal red blood cells (microcytic). Microcytic red cells form when iron availability or globin production is reduced. Iron deficiency anemia and thalassemia are common causes of microcytic anemia.

54. A: Myelodysplastic syndrome (MDS). Macrocytosis is a condition that causes the red blood cells to be larger than normal. Causes of macrocytosis include myelodysplastic syndrome (MDS), hypothyroidism, alcoholism, liver disease, and megaloblastic anemias. Anemia of inflammation and thalassemia are common causes of microcytic anemia.

55. D: Hypotension. Many of the risk factors associated with overanticoagulation in patients taking warfarin are modifiable and can decrease the patient's risk of bleeding if appropriately managed. Comorbidities such as cardiac, liver, and renal disease may affect a patient's likelihood of experiencing a supratherapeutic INR. Acute illness, variations in vitamin K intake, and medication interactions are also modifiable risk factors. Hypertension is another risk factor associated with increased bleeding risk.

56. B: 10,000. In patients with thrombocytopenia, it may be difficult to determine how low of platelet count is too low. The level at which a platelet count becomes "too low" is dependent on the underlying disorder and the individual patient. Generally speaking, a platelet count of < 50,000 is associated with a higher bleeding risk for surgical patients and a platelet count of < 10,000 is more likely to result in severe spontaneous bleeding.

57. D: Paroxysmal nocturnal hemoglobinuria (PNH). PNH is a rare disorder characterized by a variety of different potential clinical symptoms including fatigue, dyspnea, abdominal pain, hemoglobinuria, bone marrow suppression, chest pain, thrombosis, renal insufficiency, headache, and confusion. Laboratory results in PNH typically include hemolytic anemia, increased reticulocyte, lactate dehydrogenase (LDH), and bilirubin, and decreased haptoglobin.

58. B: Telangiectasia. Patients with limited cutaneous systemic sclerosis may present with CREST syndrome. CREST syndrome includes calcinosis cutis, Raynaud phenomenon, esophageal dysmotility, sclerodactyly, and telangiectasia. Telangiectasia is defined as superficial dilated blood vessels and may be present on the face and/or hands.

59. D: Secondary Sjögren syndrome. Secondary Sjögren syndrome is an inflammatory disease that occurs in patients already diagnosed with another rheumatologic disease such as rheumatoid arthritis or systemic lupus erythematosus. Symptoms of Sjögren syndrome may include dry eyes and mouth (due to decreased tear and saliva production), pain, stiffness and swelling of the joints, vasculitis, painful swelling of the salivary and parotid glands, and numbness, tingling, and weakness.

60. A: "Avoid exposure to ultraviolet light as it may exacerbate your symptoms." Exposure to ultraviolet light in patients with systemic lupus erythematosus (SLE) may exacerbate symptoms. Medications causing photosensitivity in SLE patients should also be avoided. Vitamin supplementation in patients with SLE is generally not necessary unless the patient is not eating a balanced diet. Live vaccinations such as the measles, mumps, and rubella (MMR) vaccine are contraindicated in SLE patients due to immunosuppression. Herbal supplements are not proven to provide any value in the treatment of SLE and should be avoided.

61. C: Patients with cortically located, large, multiple, and superficial-draining AVMs are more likely to present with seizures. Intracranial hemorrhage in patients with brain AVMs are more common in

children. Brain AVMs most commonly present between 10 and 40 years of age. Focal neurologic deficits are an uncommon presentation in patients with cerebral AVMs and often occur in response to hemorrhage or seizure activity. Seizure activity may occur in up to one-third of patients with brain AVMs and are more likely to occur in patients with cortically located, large, multiple, and superficial-draining AVMs.

62. B: Increased fluid in intervertebral disks. Expected physiologic musculoskeletal-related changes associated with aging include decreased bone calcium (resulting in increased osteoporosis and increased curvature of the spine), decreased fluid in intervertebral disks, decreased blood supply to muscles, decreased tissue elasticity, and decreased muscle mass.

63. D: The drugs of choice in the treatment of partial (focal) simple seizures are valproic acid and clonazepam. Partial (focal) seizures occur in only one hemisphere of the brain and can either be classified as complex or simple. Complex partial seizures are associated with a loss of consciousness and typically last 1 to 3 minutes. Simple partial seizures are typically associated with an aura and not a loss of consciousness. Preferred pharmacologic agents for the treatment of partial (focal) seizures (both simple and complex) include phenytoin and carbamazepine.

64. A: Lewy body dementia. Lewy body dementia shares many similarities with Parkinson disease, with early symptoms including parkinsonism. Other symptoms may include hallucinations, changes in thinking and reasoning, and confusion. Frontotemporal dementia is diagnosed based on changes in personality and the presence of frontal brain atrophy. Vascular dementia usually includes an abrupt onset of dementia, abnormal reflexes or nerve functions, and/or evidence of cerebrovascular accidents on imaging. Early symptoms of Alzheimer disease include memory impairment followed by impaired judgment, disorientation and confusion, and trouble speaking, swallowing, and walking.

65. B: Agnosia. Agnosia is defined as the inability to recognize objects. Agnosia can contribute to serious safety hazards such as causing patients to attempt to eat an inedible item or misuse a piece of cooking equipment in their activities of daily living. Anomia is defined as the inability to name an object and usually precedes agnosia. Apraxia is defined as the loss of ability to perform activities or the inability to carry out purposeful movements. Anhedonia is the inability to experience pleasure and is a common feature of depression.

66. C: Rupture of arterial aneurysms. Subarachnoid hemorrhage occurs when there is sudden bleeding into the subarachnoid space. This bleeding is most commonly caused by the rupture of arterial aneurysms. Thrombus formation in an artery is associated with a thrombotic stroke. Hypertension and vascular malformations are common causes of intracerebral hemorrhage.

67. D: Sepsis. Acute toxic-metabolic encephalopathy refers to a disruption in the balance of the neurological environment in which electrolytes, water, amino acids, and neurotransmitters affect the normal activity of the neurons. Symptoms include delirium and confusion, seizures, and motor abnormalities. Encephalopathy due to sepsis is the most common cause of acute toxic-metabolic encephalopathy. Increased ammonia level is associated with hepatic encephalopathy. Hypoxia is associated with hypoxic-ischemic encephalopathy. Hyponatremia is a common cause of acute toxic-metabolic encephalopathy.

68. A: < 15 mm Hg. Normal intracranial pressure in adults is < 15 mm Hg. Pathologic intracranial hypertension occurs when intracranial pressure reaches > 20 mm Hg. Elevated intracranial pressure is associated with headache, change in level of consciousness, and vomiting.

69. C: Tissue resonance analysis. Intraventricular monitoring is the gold standard for monitoring of intracranial pressure. Intraventricular monitors are surgically placed into the ventricle equipped with a pressure transducer, drainage bag, and stopcock. Epidural monitors are equipped with optical transducers and rest against the dura. The fiber optic Camino system is a type of intraparenchymal monitor equipped with a fiber optic tip and placed directly into the parenchyma of the brain. Tissue resonance analysis is a noninvasive intracranial pressure monitoring option that has been researched and showed potential promise in ICP monitoring. Results of this method, however, have been inconsistent and lacking in practical applicability. Use of tissue resonance analysis is not currently recommended in the literature.

70. B: Intracranial hypertension associated with a brain tumor. The administration of glucocorticoids are contraindicated in patients diagnosed with increased intracranial pressure due to moderate to severe head injury, intracranial hemorrhage, or cerebral infarction. Studies indicate a less favorable outcome if glucocorticoids are administered in this setting. However, glucocorticoids may be useful in the treatment of intracranial hypertension associated with brain tumors or infections of the central nervous system.

71. D: West Nile virus. Parotitis is indicative of encephalitis caused by mumps. Hydrophobia, pharyngeal spasms, and hyperactivity are associated with encephalitic rabies. Encephalitis caused by the varicella zoster virus often produces grouped vesicles along a dermatome. West Nile virus is associated with flaccid paralysis evolving into encephalitis accompanied by the presence of a maculopapular rash.

72. D: All of the above. Headaches associated with brain tumors vary in character based on tumor location, size, and rate of growth. They are frequently associated with other symptoms including seizures, fatigue, cognitive dysfunction, nausea and vomiting, and focal weakness. Both primary brain tumors and brain tumors caused by metastasis are equally likely to cause headaches.

73. B: Amyotrophic lateral sclerosis (ALS). ALS is the most common form of motor neuron disease. ALS is a progressive neuromuscular disorder characterized the combination of both upper and lower motor neuron signs and symptoms, including muscle weakness, disability, and eventual death. Muscular dystrophies are a group of progressive myopathic disorders that result from genetic defects and affect the ability of the muscles to function properly. Multiple sclerosis (MS) is most common immune-mediated inflammatory demyelinating disease of the central nervous system. Acute transverse myelitis is a rare neuroimmune spinal cord disorder characterized by rapid onset weakness and sensory alterations. Acute transverse myelitis is usually seen in conjunction with a postinfectious process.

74. C: Motor complete. The American Spinal Injury Association (ASIA) scale includes the classifications complete cord injury, sensory incomplete, motor incomplete, and normal. Complete cord injury is defined as the absence of motor or sensory function preserved in the sacral segments S4-5. Sensory incomplete is scored when sensory but not motor function is preserved below the neurologic level (includes sacral segments) and no motor function is preserved more than 3 levels below the motor level on either side. Motor incomplete may be scored as a "C" or "D" class depending on the severity. Motor incomplete "C" occurs when motor function is preserved below the neurologic level and more than half of key muscle functions below the neurologic level of injury have a muscle grade < 3 (grades 0 to 2). Motor incomplete "D" occurs when motor function is preserved below the neurologic level and at least half of key muscle functions below the neurologic

level of injury have a muscle grade ≥ 3. To be classified as normal, sensation and motor function are graded as normal in all segments with the patient having had prior defects.

75. B: Serum glucose < 70 mg/dL. Clinical exclusion criteria for the administration of recombinant tissue plasminogen activator in the treatment of acute ischemic stroke include symptoms suggestive of subarachnoid hemorrhage, persistent blood pressure elevation (SBP > 185 mm Hg or DBP > 110 mm Hg), serum glucose < 50 mg/dL, and active internal bleeding. Additionally hematologic exclusion criteria include platelet count < 100,000/mm³, current anticoagulant use with an INR > 1.7 or PT > 15 seconds, heparin use within 48 hours and an abnormally elevated aPTT, and current use of direct thrombin inhibitor or direct factor Xa inhibitor with evidence of anticoagulation.

76. C: Liver and pancreas lab tests are typically abnormal. Functional gallbladder disease is defined as a motility disorder of the gallbladder that may be caused by a primary motility disorder or metabolic disorder. Patients typically present with biliary colic. Liver function and pancreatic enzymes are typically normal with the absence of gallstones or sludge on imaging. Endoscopic examinations of the upper gastrointestinal tract are also normal in patients with functional gallbladder disease. Patients with functional gallbladder disorder are candidates for cholecystectomy if biliary colic is present with the ejection fraction of the gallbladder being less than 40%.

77. C: Weight loss. According to the Rome III criteria, dyspepsia is defined as early satiation, epigastric pain, and postprandial fullness. Dyspepsia may be caused by a variety of disease processes including (but not limited to) gastroesophageal reflux disease (GERD), gastric and esophageal malignancy, gastroparesis, pancreatitis, medications, Crohn disease, sarcoidosis, metabolic disturbances, and intestinal parasites. Weight loss may be a symptom of an underlying disease (such as malignancy) that may emerge as the disease progresses.

78. D: All of the above. There are several known factors that may increase a person's risk of developing colorectal cancer. They include increasing age, a diet high in fat, a diet high in red or processed meat and low in fiber, sedentary lifestyle, smoking, alcohol use, and obesity. In addition, familial adenomatous polyposis, hereditary nonpolyposis or Lynch syndrome, and inflammatory bowel disease greatly increase risk. Increased calcium intake, use of nonsteroidal anti-inflammatory drugs, and use of aspirin may be associated with a decreased risk of colorectal cancer.

79. C: Gastroparesis. The presence of abdominal pain with vomiting may be indicative of cholelithiasis. Symptoms of intestinal obstruction include feculent vomiting. Acute viral gastroenteritis symptoms include nausea, vomiting, diarrhea, fever, and abdominal pain. Vomiting of food eaten several hours earlier and the presence of succussion splash on abdominal auscultation may indicate gastroparesis or gastric obstruction.

80. B: 5-HT$_3$ receptor antagonists. 5-HT$_3$ receptor antagonists are the most useful antiemetic agents for patients with chemotherapy-induced emesis. Agents include ondansetron, granisetron, dolasetron, and palonosetron. These agents are generally well tolerated with the most frequent side effect being headache.

81. D: Extrapyramidal reactions. Extrapyramidal (EPS) reactions are a relatively common side effect of phenothiazines. EPS reactions may include dystonia, and tardive dyskinesia with prolonged administration. Hypotension may also occur, more commonly in older adults. Abdominal pain and headache are rare side effects of phenothiazines.

82. A: Mallory-Weiss tear. Mallory-Weiss tears occur when mucosal lacerations form in the distal esophagus and proximal stomach, which often lead to bleeding from the submucosal arteries. Emesis, retching, and coughing prior to hematemesis are symptoms indicative of a Mallory-Weiss tear. Mallory-Weiss tears account for approximately 5% of all patient presenting with upper gastrointestinal bleeding. Dysphagia, early satiety, unintentional weight loss, and cachexia are symptoms associated with malignancy. Patients with peptic ulcers may present with epigastric or right upper quadrant abdominal pain in addition to the bleeding. Esophageal ulcer symptoms may include dysphagia and gastroesophageal reflux.

83. C: Elevated platelet count. Acute liver failure occurs when there is evidence of severe liver injury resulting in encephalopathy and impaired synthetic function (thereby affecting coagulation). Hepatic encephalopathy, elevated aminotransferase levels, and prolonged prothrombin time are all diagnostic criteria for acute liver failure. Platelets are typically decreased in patients with acute liver failure.

84. D: Spleen and liver. Blunt abdominal trauma commonly occurs in patients who have experienced a motor vehicle accident. Blunt abdominal trauma accounts for a large percentage of patients presenting to the emergency department with abdominal injury. The spleen and liver are the most commonly injured solid organs in blunt abdominal trauma. Injuries to the pancreas, bowel, diaphragm, bladder, kidneys, and abdominal aorta are less common.

85. C: Patients with acute hepatitis C infection typically have serum aminotransferase levels that are moderately to highly elevated. Patients with acute hepatitis C infection are typically asymptomatic. Of those who are symptomatic, jaundice, dark urine, nausea, and abdominal pain are common symptoms. Serum aminotransferase levels are typically moderately to highly elevated with values often 10 to 20 times greater than the upper limit of normal. Acute illness typically lasts for 2 to 12 weeks. Fulminant hepatic failure in patients with acute hepatitis C infection is rare.

86. A: International travel. Hepatitis A infection is caused by a viral infection (hepatitis A virus) resulting in acute hepatitis. Hepatitis A is spread via the fecal-oral route. The most common risk factor for hepatitis A in the United States is international travel, accounting for approximately 50% of all hepatitis A infections in the United States. Other risk factors include sexual or household contact with an infected person, homosexual activity in men, food or waterborne exposure, resident or employee of a daycare center or group home, and injection drug use.

87. C: Steatorrhea. Clinical findings characterizing chronic pancreatitis include diabetes mellitus, pancreatic calculi, pain, and steatorrhea. A decrease in the enzymes lipase and protease results in steatorrhea, the presence of excess fat in the stool. Pain is the most common clinical finding, with 90% to 95% of patients with chronic pancreatitis experiencing it. Pain associated with chronic pancreatitis is epigastric in nature, often radiating to the back.

88. A: Inflammatory bowel disease. Inflammatory bowel disease causes inflammation of the gastrointestinal tract, leading to nausea, pain, fever, and diarrhea. These symptoms eventually lead to loss of appetite and impaired nutritional status. Inflammatory bowel disease is associated with the depletion of muscle and fat. It is less commonly associated with weight loss and protein calorie malnutrition.

89. D: Nonsteroidal anti-inflammatory drugs. Perforation can occur when diverticula are present in the small intestine, duodenum, or colon. Diverticular perforations may also lead to the formation of

an abscess. Nonsteroidal anti-inflammatory drugs and glucocorticoids are the 2 classes of medications that are associated with an increased risk of diverticular perforation. Diverticular perforations may also lead to the formation of an abscess.

90. C: Metronidazole. Antibiotic therapy altering the normal flora of the gastrointestinal tract is the mechanism by which *Clostridium difficile* is able to colonize, resulting in the development of a pseudomembranous colitis. Metronidazole is the drug of choice for first line therapy in the treatment of non-severe *C. difficile* infection. Oral vancomycin may also be used in the initial treatment of non-severe *C. difficile*. Metronidazole is preferred over vancomycin as it is less costly and limits the spread of vancomycin resistant enterococci. Fidaxomicin and rifaximin are agents that may be utilized in recurrent *C. difficile* infections or in conjunction with other agents.

91. B: Isotonic saline. Patients with acute kidney injury often experience volume depletion and may present with signs and symptoms of hypovolemia (hypotension and tachycardia) and oliguria. Intravenous fluid replacement is indicated in volume-depleted patients, with the preferred choice for initial therapy being crystalloid fluids. Colloid fluids (such as Hespan) may also be used, but they are more costly than crystalloid fluids and have proven to offer no additional benefit. Potassium-containing fluids such as lactated Ringer's should be avoided in the patient with acute kidney injury as it may cause hyperkalemia.

92. B: 3 months. Chronic kidney disease occurs when kidney damage or decreased kidney function is present for 3 or more months, regardless of the cause. Chronic kidney disease is staged according to cause, albuminuria, and estimated glomerular filtration rate (eGFR). Acute kidney injury is defined as the abrupt loss of kidney function.

93. D: Bladder outlet obstruction. Overflow incontinence in women is often caused by underactivity of the detrusor muscle (due to impaired contractility) and bladder outlet obstruction (due to compression of the urethra). Intrinsic sphincteric deficiency and urethral hypermobility are associated with stress incontinence. Overactive bladder (urgency incontinence) is associated with increasing age and overactivity of the detrusor muscle.

94. C: *Escherichia coli*. Catheter-associated urinary tract infections (CAUTI) are a common cause of healthcare-associated infections, accounting for more than 30% of hospital-acquired infections. *Escherichia coli* is the most common organism associated with catheter-associated urinary tract infections. Other common organisms associated with CAUTI are *Candida*, *Enterococcus*, *Pseudomonas aeruginosa*, *Klebsiella pneumoniae*, and *Enterobacter*.

95. C: Orange juice. Decreased fluid intake is associated with an increased risk of kidney stone formation. The types of fluid that people ingest may also be significant. Orange juice (containing both potassium and citrate) is associated with a decreased risk of crystal formation. This may be related to increased urinary citrate excretion. Sugar-sweetened drinks have been linked to an increased risk of kidney stone formation. Cranberry juice has not been associated with either an increased or decreased risk of stone formation.

96. D: Right upper quadrant pain with referred right shoulder pain. Women with symptomatic pelvic inflammatory disease typically present with abnormal uterine bleeding (menorrhagia or postcoital bleeding), lower abdominal pain, and purulent endocervical or vaginal discharge. Perihepatitis occurs in approximately 10% of women with pelvic inflammatory disease. Inflammation of the liver results in right upper quadrant pain with a pleuritic component, often causing a referred right shoulder pain.

97. A: *Chlamydia trachomatis*. In female patients younger than 25 years, annually screening for *Chlamydia trachomatis* and *Neisseria gonorrhoeae* is recommended. Additionally, screening for HIV is recommended once (more frequently in high-risk patients). Routine screening for *Mycoplasma genitalium* is not recommended. Routine screening for syphilis is also not recommended for asymptomatic patients.

98. D: Hypocalcemia. Hypocalcemia may occur in patients with malignancy, chronic malabsorption syndrome, hyperphosphatemia, excessive GI losses of calcium, and diuretic use. Signs and symptoms may include dysrhythmias, lethargy, tonic/clonic seizures, constipation, muscle cramps or tremors, bone pain, and oliguria. Hypocalcemia is diagnosed by a serum calcium level. Other indications of hypocalcemia include Trousseau sign and Chvostek sign. Treatment includes the replacement of calcium with calcium gluconate or calcium chloride. Vitamin D may also be administered.

99. D: Salt craving. Hypovolemia due to volume depletion may result in a variety of symptoms including physical symptoms and laboratory abnormalities. Early symptoms include thirst, muscle cramps, postural dizziness, lack of energy, and easy fatigability. Oliguria may also be present. Salt craving is a symptom that occurs in patients with primary adrenal insufficiency.

100. C: Class III. Surgical wounds or incisions are made during a surgical procedure in a sterile, controlled environment. The American College of Surgeons has defined 4 classes of surgical wound types. This classification can help to predict how the wound will heal and the risk of infection. Class I is defined as clean (examples include laparoscopic surgeries and biopsies), class II is defined as clean contaminated (examples include GI and GU surgeries), class III is defined as contaminated (example includes traumatic wounds such as a gunshot wound), and class IV is defined as dirty (example includes traumatic wound from a dirty source).

101. B: Collagenase. Enzymatic debridement therapy may be utilized as a treatment option for patients who are not candidates for surgical debridement. Collagenase is an enzymatic debriding agent approved for the debridement of chronic wounds and burns. Chlorhexidine is an antiseptic solution typically not used in the irrigation of wounds. Becaplermin is a platelet-derived growth factor used to promote angiogenesis. Cadexomer iodine is an iodine-based antimicrobial topical preparation used in the treatment of wounds.

102. A: Pallor and pulselessness are early signs of compartment syndrome. Compartment syndrome occurs when there is an increase in the amount of pressure within a grouping of muscles, nerves, and blood vessels resulting in compromised blood flow to muscles and nerves. If left untreated, tissue ischemia and eventual tissue death will occur. Compartment syndrome most often occurs after a fracture, particularly a long bone fracture. Risk factors for the development of compartment syndrome also include lower extremity trauma, massive tissue injury, venous obstruction, the use of certain medications (anticoagulants), burns, and compressive dressings or casts. Compartment syndrome can also occur with crush syndrome and rhabdomyolysis. Compartment syndrome can affect the hand, forearm, upper arm, abdomen, and lower extremities. It can be acute or chronic in nature with acute compartment syndrome requiring immediate intervention. Signs and symptoms include intense pain, decreased sensation and paresthesia, firmness at the affected site, swelling and tightness at the affected site, pallor, and pulselessness (late signs). The goal of treatment in compartment syndrome is decompression and the restoration of perfusion to the affected area. Often, surgical fasciotomy is indicated to relieve pressure and prevent tissue death. Fasciotomy

involves the opening of the skin and muscle fascia to release the pressure within the compartment and restore blood flow to the area.

103. D: 48 hours. Ventilator-associated events (VAE) include a broad range of complications that may occur in the ventilated patient. Aspiration is a potential complication of intubation and greatly increases the risk of developing VAE in the critical care patient. Ventilator-associated pneumonia (VAP) is a healthcare-associated infection that develops in a patient with an endotracheal tube or tracheostomy who has been mechanically ventilated for at least 48 hours when the infection is identified. Risk factors for the development of VAP include advanced age, immobility, postoperative patients, and immunocompromised patients.

104. D: A severe alteration in consciousness with intermittent demonstration of restricted purposeful behavior and following commands. Minimally conscious state (MCS) is a term used to describe patients who do not meet the criteria for persistent vegetative state. Patients with MCS have a severe alteration in consciousness but may exhibit intermittent demonstration of restricted purposeful behavior or following of commands. No evidence of awareness of self or environment and inability to interact with others is associated with a persistent vegetative state. Locked-in syndrome is defined by awakeness and alertness with the inability to move or communicate due to paralysis of muscles. Brain death is associated with no respiratory drive or ability to spontaneously breathe.

105. A: Disability. The ABCD prioritization model or survey is an assessment tool often used by first-line responders to assess a trauma patient and prioritize treatment. Airway, Breathing, Circulation, and Disability define the model. In assessing for disability, a rapid neurological assessment should be conducted to assess the level and severity of injury.

106. C: The wound is superficial with partial thickness skin loss involving the epidermis or dermis. A staging system (consisting of 4 stages) is useful in characterizing the damage caused by pressure ulcers. Stage 1 is defined as skin intact with no evidence of pressure changes. In stage 2 pressure ulcers, the wound is superficial with partial thickness skin loss involving the epidermis or dermis. Stage 3 ulcers have full thickness skin loss extending into the subcutaneous tissue. In stage 4 ulcers, extensive destruction is evident, including damage to muscle, bone, or supporting structures.

107. D: *Klebsiella pneumoniae*. Carbapenem-resistant *Enterobacteriaceae* (CRE) are a family of resistant organisms that were formerly susceptible to the antibiotic class carbapenems. The majority of CRE infections are caused by the *Klebsiella pneumoniae* organism. CRE infections are associated with an increased mortality rate and are more likely to occur in hospitalized patients who are mechanically ventilated, have an indwelling intravenous or urinary catheter, or have received a long-term course of antibiotic therapy.

108. B: The use of bone-modifying agents to prevent skeletal events including fractures and bone pain caused by bone metastases. The use of bone-modifying agents is considered standard treatment in patients with lytic bone lesions. The use of these agents can prevent skeletal fractures and bone pain caused by metastasis. Bisphosphonates inhibit osteoclast-mediated bone resorption. Patients should be educated on taking analgesics around the clock to prevent pain. According to the World Health Organization 3-step analgesic ladder, adjuvant agents should be used to treat symptoms associated with pain such as anxiety or depression. Pharmacologic management of pain should begin with nonopioid therapy and progress to the use of opioids when pain persists or increases.

109. D: All of the above. Palliative sedation is defined as the use of pharmacologic agents to provide a state of decreased consciousness with the intent of limiting suffering associated with intractable symptoms in the imminently dying patient. All available pharmacologic and psychosocial treatments should be utilized prior to the implementation of palliative sedation. Palliative care specialists should be consulted to ensure that all available treatment options have been exhausted for the intractable symptom(s).

110. A: A patient who states it is painful to brush her hair. Allodynia is defined as a painful response to a normally innocuous stimulus, such as brushing one's hair or shaving one's face. Dysesthesia is defined as a spontaneous or evoked unpleasant and abnormal sensation. This can include burning, tingling, and the sensation of being on fire. Hyperalgesia is an increased response to a noxious stimulus. Hyperalgesia is common in opioid withdrawal. Prolonged pain after a transient stimulus is defined as persistent pain.

111. D: All of the above. Respiratory distress is commonly experienced in the dying patient and may be exceptionally distressing to the patient and their family. Palliative treatment options include the administration of opioids, the drug of choice in end-of-life dyspnea. Supplemental oxygen may provide comfort and decrease hypoxemia. Atropine may be administered to help decrease bronchial secretions that contribute to distress.

112. D: The administration of medication to relieve pain even if the unintended consequence is hastening of death by respiratory depression. The principle of double effect is defined as a mechanism to provide permissibility of an action that may result in an adverse outcome or serious harm in an attempt to do good. In palliative care, the administration of medication to relieve pain to relieve suffering may result in the unintended consequence of hastening death through respiratory depression. The correlated action of two or more medications is known as synergy. The enhancement of the effect of a drug, treatment, or biologic is defined as adjuvant therapy. The intentional, painless ending of life of a patient suffering from an incurable and painful disease is euthanasia.

113. B: Methotrexate. Extravasation occurs when an intravenously infused vesicant medication or fluid leaks from the vein and into the subcutaneous space. Vesicant medications are those that cause tissue injury if extravasated and that may ultimately lead to tissue necrosis. Extravasation and infiltration are similar in nature, with infiltration occurring when the infusate is a nonvesicant solution or medication. Extravasation occurs more commonly in peripheral IVs; however, it can also occur with central venous catheters. Common vesicant agents include several chemotherapeutic agents, vancomycin, electrolytes, dobutamine, norepinephrine, phenytoin, promethazine, propofol and vasopressin. Methotrexate is classified as a nonvesicant agent.

114. A: Auditory nerve damage. Conductive hearing loss is related to an impedance of external sound gaining access to the inner ear. Potential causes of conductive hearing loss include lack of movement of small bones of the inner ear, fluid in the middle ear, or cerumen impaction. Auditory nerve, inner ear, or cochlear impairments are related to sensorineural hearing loss.

115. C: Weber and Rinne test. Weber and Rinne tests are not utilized as a screening tool for evaluation of hearing loss, but rather as a means to differentiate between conductive and sensorineural hearing loss. Pneumoscopy is a test used to evaluate the mobility of the tympanic membrane in patients with conductive hearing loss. An audiogram may be conducted on patients

without a known etiology for their hearing loss. CT scan of the temporal bone may be performed in patients with unexplained conductive hearing loss.

116. B: Increased length of stay. The Nurses Improving Care of Healthsystem Elders (NICHE) program was initiated in the early 1990s in an effort to improve the care of the elderly hospitalized patient. Studies have shown that hospitals that have adopted the NICHE program have made an impact on the care of the hospitalized elderly patient through fall reduction, decreased restraint use, decreased confusion, decreased hospital acquired infections, decreased length of stay, and decreased costs.

117. D: Serum salicylate 45 mg/dL. Salicylate toxicity can occur in adult patients after the ingestion of 10 to 30 grams of salicylates. Therapeutic serum salicylate levels fall between 10 mg/dL and 30 mg/dL. Values exceeding 40 mg/dL are associated with toxicity. Salicylate toxicity may cause nausea, vomiting, diarrhea, tinnitus, vertigo, pulmonary edema, changes in mental status, coma, and death.

118. D: Serum lead level. Clinical manifestations of lead poisoning include abdominal pain, headache, joint pain, extreme fatigue, irritability, decreased libido, sleep disturbances, constipation, and anemia. High lead levels may result in peripheral neuropathy, confusion, seizures, and encephalopathy. Patients at risk of lead poisoning include those who work in the manufacturing or use of batteries, pigments, solder, ammunitions, paint, car radiators, cable and wires, ceramic ware with lead glazes, and tin cans. In addition, lead smelting and refinement may also contribute to exposure.

119. B: Lactate > 2 mmol/L after adequate fluid resuscitation. Septic shock is a vasodilatory type of shock manifested by a lactate level > 2 mmol/L and the required use of vasopressors to maintain a mean arterial pressure of > 65 mm Hg despite adequate fluid resuscitation. Septic shock is associated with a higher mortality rate than sepsis alone. Clinical manifestations of sepsis are somewhat nonspecific but may include a temperature of > 38.3 degrees Celsius, a white blood cell count > 12,000, tachypnea, tachycardia, arterial hypotension, and altered mental status.

120. D: Lactic acid. The sequential organ failure assessment is a tool that may be utilized to predict ICU mortality in patients with multiorgan dysfunction syndrome (MODS). The scale includes platelet count, partial pressure of arterial oxygen ($PaO_2$)/fraction of inspired oxygen ($FiO_2$) ratio, serum bilirubin, serum creatinine or urine output, hypotension and vasopressor requirement, and Glasgow coma scale.

121. D: Core temperature of > 38 degrees Celsius. Systemic inflammatory response syndrome (SIRS) occurs when tissues distant from the original source of insult to the body begin to show signs of inflammation, resulting in vasodilation and accumulation of leukocytes. Defining characteristics of SIRS include core temperature of > 38.5°C or < 36°C, tachycardia, defined as a mean heart rate more than 2 standard deviations above normal for age, mean respiratory rate more than 2 standard deviations above normal for age or mechanical ventilation for an acute pulmonary process, and leukocyte count elevated or depressed for age (or > 10% immature neutrophils).

122. D: Serotonin norepinephrine reuptake inhibitors. Serotonin norepinephrine reuptake inhibitors are a class of medications traditionally used to treat major depression and anxiety. They have also shown to be effective in the treatment of diabetic peripheral neuropathy, fibromyalgia, chronic lower back pain, and osteoarthritis. Venlafaxine, desvenlafaxine, duloxetine, and milnacipran are the serotonin norepinephrine reuptake inhibitors available in the United States.

123. C: "I would like to start your mother on some acetaminophen for her osteoarthritis pain. We will see if this is effective over the next couple of days and if not we can make some modifications to her pain management regimen." Elderly patients with dementia can accurately and reliably report pain. Recommendations in the treatment of elderly patients with dementia who are experiencing pain include a prescribed trial of scheduled analgesics and cautious monitoring and weighing risks and benefits of treatment. Starting with a low dose and progressing slowly is also recommended. Opioids are not a first choice for treatment in elderly patients, especially in the opioid-naïve patient. Glucosamine and chondroitin, although they have shown some effectiveness in the management of osteoarthritis-related pain, are not recommended treatment options.

124. B: Rivastigmine. Neuropsychiatric symptoms are commonly experienced in patients with dementia and may include agitation, aggression, hallucinations, delusions, and depression. Benzodiazepines are not recommended in the treatment of neuropsychiatric symptoms. Antihistamines are also not recommended due to the high incidence of side effects. Cholinesterase inhibitors are recommended for patients with mild to moderate dementia who are experiencing neuropsychiatric symptoms. They are generally well tolerated and may also assist with cognition and functional ability.

125. C: Minimize cognitive stimulation. Delirium is defined as an acute state of confusion precipitated by an underlying physiological condition or effect of a medication. Strategies to mitigate the risk of developing delirium include orientation of the patient to their environment, facilitation of sleep and minimization of sleep interruptions, early mobilization, promotion of cognitive stimulation (using caution to not overly stimulate), and the avoidance of medications that may precipitate delirium.

126. B: Dehydration. Failure to thrive in elderly patients is defined by 3 components: disability, impaired neuropsychiatric function, and physical frailty. Physical frailty includes weight loss, malnutrition, and physical inactivity. Disability involves difficulty in the completion of activities of daily living. Impairment of neuropsychiatric function may include delirium, dementia, and depression.

127. A: Loss of weight. The FRAIL scale is a mnemonic that can be utilized to assess an elderly patient for frailty. A yes to 3 or more of the questions confirms the presence of frailty. F-fatigue R-resistance A-ambulation I-illness L-loss of weight. Loss of weight is defined as weight loss of > 5%.

128. C: The highest rates of elder abuse are in women. Elder abuse and mistreatment is often underreported and therefore clinicians should conduct appropriate screenings and assessments to recognize abuse. Warning signs may be present including skin conditions (eg, tears, pressure ulcers, lacerations, bruises), malnutrition, dehydration, and fractures. Elder mistreatment may also involve the administration of inappropriate mediations or the administration of incorrect medication doses. The abuser is often a family member (90% of the time).

129. A: Selective serotonin reuptake inhibitor (SSRI). Obsessive-compulsive disorder is a psychiatric disorder that is characterized by obsessions (recurrent intrusive thoughts or images) or compulsions (repetitive mental or behavioral acts) or both. Front-line therapy includes cognitive behavioral therapy and, for patients who require pharmacologic therapy, an SSRI.

130. D: Intravitreal bevacizumab. Age-related macular degeneration is a common cause of visual impairment in adults. There are 2 types of macular degeneration: dry type and wet type. In wet

macular degeneration, abnormal blood vessels grow under the retina and macula. This results in leakage of fluid that ultimately distorts the macula, resulting in rapid and severe vision loss. Intravitreal administration of vascular endothelial growth factors (such as bevacizumab) may be utilized to slow progression and even help to reverse vision loss. Topical prostaglandins and topical beta-blockers are indicated in the treatment of open-angle glaucoma. Intraocular lens implantation may be indicated in the treatment of cataracts.

131. D: Notify Mr. Jones' family that he is not competent to care for himself or make health care decisions based on his nonadherence. Medical nonadherence is defined by the World Health Organization as "the extent to which a person's behavior corresponds with agreed upon recommendations from a health care provider." Recommendations may include medications, diet, and other lifestyle modifications. Nonadherence with treatment regimens significantly contributes to hospital readmissions in patients with chronic diseases. It is also one of the most common causes of treatment failure. There are many potential reasons why patient do not adhere to the recommendations of their health care provider. Factors may include the perception that the prescribed treatment is ineffective, the treatment has adverse or unpleasant effects, or the cost of the treatment is too high. In addition, the patient may not fully understand the importance of the prescribed treatment or may forget to take medications as prescribed. The patient may encounter barriers that make the necessary lifestyle modifications difficult. Simplifying medication regimens and ensuring the patient has a thorough understanding of the prescribed treatment plan is critical in promoting adherence. Enlisting the support of family and friends and involving the patient and the family in the plan of care is also important. Discharge instructions should be written in terms that the patient understands and an assessment of the patient's level of understanding should be performed. Follow-up phone calls may also be helpful in promoting adherence.

132. C: Elderly white men 85 years and older. The risk of suicide increases with age, with elderly white men 85 years and older having the highest suicide rate in the United States. However, younger adults attempt suicide more frequently. Females attempt suicide more frequently than males; however, males complete suicide more frequently than females. Suicide rates are higher amongst whites than African Americans but in recent years suicide rates have increased amongst young African-American males.

133. A: Patients should not be questioned about suicidal thoughts by clinicians as this may prompt the patient to experience suicidal thoughts or actions. Patients determined to be at risk for suicide should be questioned about suicidal ideation. Psychiatric disorders, previous suicide attempts, and feelings of hopelessness are major risk factors for suicide. Questioning patients regarding suicidal ideation has not been proven to increase one's risk of suicide or promote suicidal ideation. Social and family support helps to decrease the risk of suicide.

134. C: Ask, Advise, Assess, Assist, Arrange. Smoking is a leading cause of preventable mortality, with up to 70% of smokers expressing a desire to quit. The five A's algorithm was developed as a tool to assess for tobacco use and to address smoking cessation. The algorithm includes asking about tobacco status, advising tobacco users to quit smoking, assessing the patient's willingness to quit, assisting by providing the patient with aids to quit smoking, and arranging follow-up contact.

135. D: All of the above. In addition to pharmacologic treatment options for smoking cessation, nonpharmacologic treatment options exist that may be effective. Behavioral counseling has been shown to increase cessation rates and may be available to patients in different formats, including smoking cessation programs, computer-based programs, and one-on-one counseling. Acupuncture

and hypnosis are other nonpharmacologic treatment options that may or may not be effective in smoking cessation, as efficacy has not been proven.

136. B: Female gender. Obstructive sleep apnea is the most common sleep-related breathing disorder. Risk factors for obstructive sleep apnea include advanced age, male gender, craniofacial or soft tissue abnormalities in the upper airway, and obesity. Obesity is the strongest risk factor for the development of obstructive sleep apnea. Smoking, menopause, and family history of obstructive sleep apnea are additional risk factors.

137. D: "I will have a colonoscopy every 3 years as part of my screening for colon cancer." According to the US Preventive Services Task Force (USPSTF) recommendations, colon cancer screening should begin at age 50. For patients with a close relative with colorectal polyps or colorectal cancer, patients with inflammatory bowel disease, or patients with a familial adenomatous polyposis (FAP), screening may be recommended at an earlier age. Screening can be performed using high-sensitivity fecal occult blood testing (recommend yearly testing), sigmoidoscopy (recommend every 5 years or if performed in combination with high-sensitivity fecal occult blood testing every 3 years), or colonoscopy (recommend every 10 years).

138. C: Transfused blood cells are broken down and destroyed days or weeks after the transfusion. Delayed hemolytic blood transfusion reactions occur when the body slowly attacks the non-ABO antigens on the transfused blood cells. This occurs days or weeks after the transfusion. Patients do not usually experience any symptoms. This type of reaction occurs in patients who have previously received blood products. The transfused blood cells are destroyed and the patient's red blood cell count falls.

139. E: A, B, D. Mannitol is an osmotic diuretic that may be administered to treat increased intracranial pressure (ICP) and reduce cerebral edema. Mannitol is considered a vesicant and care must be taken to avoid extravasation. It is recommended that mannitol be administered via a large peripheral vein or central vein when possible. Each dose should be given over 20 to 30 minutes; rapid infusion can cause harm to the patient. Crystals may form within the IV solution; therefore, mannitol must be administered using a filter. Mannitol is contraindicated for patients with severe heart failure as the expansion of extracellular fluid can aggravate cardiac decompensation.

140. D: Cytomegalovirus increases the risk of renal cell carcinoma. Colonization of the stomach with *Helicobacter pylori* is a cause of gastric cancer and gastric mucosa-associated lymphoid (MALT) lymphoma. The most common risk factor for liver cancer is chronic infection with hepatitis B or hepatitis C. High-risk human papillomaviruses (HPVs) account for 5% of cancers worldwide. HPV is associated with cervical, vaginal, vulvar, penile, and anal cancers. It has been hypothesized that cytomegalovirus may be associated with breast cancer and brain cancer progression; however, a confirmed link has not been established. There is no correlation between cytomegalovirus and renal cell carcinoma.

141. A: The clinical skills/professional behaviors of a clinician that focus on the cultural beliefs, values, and perceptions of the patient during the therapeutic relationship established between the patient and clinician. Culturally competent care includes the recognition of an individual's cultural beliefs, values, and perceptions. According to nurse theorist Madeleine Leininger, culturally competent healthcare providers possess the clinical skills and professional behaviors that allow them to assist and support their patients in retaining and/or preserving relevant care values so that they may maintain well-being and recover from illness. Culture is defined as a way of life belonging to an individual or group of individuals that reflects values and customs. Diversity is the recognition

that each individual is unique along the dimensions of race, gender, ethnicity, religious beliefs, and sexual orientation. Cultural appropriation is the adoption of the elements of one culture by members of a different culture.

142. C: Cultural imposition. Cultural imposition occurs when an individual or group attempts to impose their values and beliefs on another individual. Cultural competence occurs when clinicians assist and support their patients in retaining and/or preserving relevant care values. Cultural blindness occurs when a person adopts or follows cultural norms of a particular culture without knowing if it is right or wrong. Ethnocentrism is defined as the belief that one's own ethnic group is superior to other ethnic groups.

143. B: Cultural pain. When a patient experiences a lack of cultural sensitivity or cultural imposition from their healthcare provider, cultural pain may occur. According to nursing theorist Madeline Leininger, cultural pain refers to the suffering and discomfort that a patient may experience when an individual or group show a lack of sensitivity towards another culture." Acculturation refers to the modification of one's culture by adapting to the traits of another culture. Cultural blindness occurs when a person adopts or follows cultural norms of a particular culture without knowing if it is right or wrong. Culture shock occurs when an individual experiences disorientation, confusion or anxiety when subjected to unfamiliar cultures.

144. D: All of the above. Culturally competent care includes a heightened awareness and recognition of a patient's cultural beliefs, values, and traditions, and incorporation of those beliefs, values, and traditions into their care. Culturally competent practitioners can assist, support, and facilitate care that helps patients retain and preserve their own cultural beliefs and values during the healing process.

145. D: Utilize short, simple sentences and summarize key points at the end of a section. Low health literacy is fairly common among people of all ages, ethnicities, backgrounds, and educational levels. Written healthcare educational materials for patients should take this into consideration. Short, simple sentences should be utilized with a summarization of key points at the end of each section. Medical terms should include a brief explanation of the meaning. Graphics may be used but only if they provide clarity to the content. Printed material should be written at a fifth-grade level to promote a greater level of understanding. Geriatric patients may need larger font in printed materials. Blues, greens, and lavenders are difficult for older adults to differentiate and should be avoided.

146. C: Beneficence. Beneficence is defined as the principle of doing good. It is an essential component of patient advocacy and requires a knowledge of the cultural beliefs and values of the patient. Justice is defined as the obligation to treat everyone fairly and equally. Nonmaleficence is an ethical principle that requires clinicians to do no harm. Autonomy provides a patient the right to make their own decisions.

147. D: Autonomy. Autonomy is defined as a patient's right to make his or her own decisions. A patient's right to autonomy in healthcare decisions is recognized in the 14th amendment of the US Constitution, as well as the Patient Self-Determination Act of 1990 that states that competent individuals have the right to make their wishes known regarding end-of-life and advanced directives. Beneficence is defined as the principle of doing good. Justice is defined as the obligation to treat everyone fairly and equally. Nonmaleficence is defined as doing no harm.

148. B: Patient Self-Determination Act. The Health Insurance Portability and Accountability Act (HIPAA) was designed to protect patient privacy, confidentiality, and security of patient information. The Oregon Death with Dignity Act allows terminally ill residents of Oregon to obtain prescription medication for self-administration in order to end their life. The Genetic Information Nondiscrimination Act was passed to prevent discrimination for health insurance and employment purposes.

149. D: All of the above. Patient rights are defined as basic rules of conduct between patients and clinicians. Many healthcare organizations have a list of patient rights and responsibilities that are provided to a patient upon entrance to a healthcare facility. Many patient rights are governed by federal and/or state law and regulatory bodies. Examples of patient's rights include a patient's right to pain management, a patient's right to receive information in a manner he or she can understand, and a patient's right to participate in the development and implementation of his or her plan of care.

150. B: Arrange a family meeting with the patient and his son, along with the palliative care team, to discuss his plan of care. Advocacy opportunities commonly present themselves in end-of-life care. Patients at the end of life often feel powerless, helpless, dependent, and vulnerable. Advanced practice nurses should advocate for appropriate and compassionate end-of-life care that is in accordance with the patient's wishes. They can assist patients and families in understanding their disease and options for end-of-life care. Hospital ethics committees and consultants may be utilized if a resolution cannot be reached. These types of committees provide guidance to patients, families, and healthcare providers when ethical dilemmas arise.

151. A: Differentiate between relevant and irrelevant data. The application of critical thinking skills to the assessment phase of the nursing process includes the collection of relevant patient data, a differentiation of relevant and irrelevant data, and validation of the data. Organization and categorization of the data into patterns or groups are associated with the diagnosis phase of the nursing process. Patient progress and revision of the plan of care are critical thinking skills/tasks associated with the evaluation phase of the nursing process.

152. D: An analysis of the relationships between a system's parts in an effort to view the system holistically and explain its behavior. Systems thinking is a way of thinking that includes an analysis of the relationships between a system's parts in an effort to see and understand the system as a whole. Critical thinking is defined as the analysis and evaluation of information, beliefs, and knowledge. Convergent thinking involves limiting the number of choices or possibilities. Analytical thinking involves the breaking down of a complex problem into single components.

153. D: All of the above. Systems thinking in nursing involves an understanding of how the complexity of the healthcare system affects the care of the individual patient. Application of systems thinking in nursing has the potential to mitigate errors, improve prioritization and delegation, enhance problem solving and decision making, and enhance quality improvement initiatives.

154. A: Systems thinking cannot be measured. Systems thinking is a necessary skill for nurses. It is often utilized in quality improvement initiatives and an increase in the application of systems thinking by nurses has the potential to mitigate errors and enhance quality initiatives. Systems thinking links a person's environment to his/her behavior. Valid and reliable tools are available to measure systems thinking in an effort to improve systems thinking over time.

155. D: All of the above. There are many different approaches and strategies that can be utilized to assist nurses in learning about systems thinking. Root cause analysis is a strategy used to examine system factors that may have contributed to an error. Case studies involving human error may also be utilized to facilitate learning about systems thinking. Creation of a flowchart or process map may be helpful in increasing staff knowledge of system factors and how they relate to the process being examined.

156. D: All of the above. Malcolm Knowles' theory of adult learning is often utilized in the planning, developing, and implementing of educational programs aimed at the adult learner. His theory is based on the principle that adult learners need motivation and relevance to maximize learning effectiveness. Adults are independent, autonomous learners who are goal oriented. They want active participation in learning activities and build on past experiences in their lives.

157. A: Do not wait until the end of the presentation to address questions. Answer questions throughout the presentation. When planning a group educational session for geriatric patients, it is important to consider the learning needs of the group. Ensure that the learning environment is conducive to learning. Make sure that the presentation is not too long. Ensure enough time for questions and do not wait until the end of the presentation to answer questions. Ensure that frequent breaks are built into the time frame. Handouts or other useful items that reinforce the topic are also helpful. Teach back technique is a good strategy to use when teaching individual patients.

158. D: All of the above. Barriers to learning can include cognitive, affective, sensory, psychomotor, physical, and physiologic limitations. Examples of physical and physiologic changes that may impede an older adult's ability to learn include depression, dementia, chronic illness, pain, fatigue, decreased reflexes, impaired vision, impaired hearing, and limited mobility and range of motion.

159. D: The unique characteristics of teaching and learning of adults. The term androgogy describes the characteristics associated with teaching and learning of adults. A paradigm is a theory or group of ideas about how something should be done. Literacy is an individual's ability to read and write. Gerogogy is the process of stimulating and helping older people learn.

160. D: All of the above. It is important for the advanced practice nurse to consider a patient's learning needs as well as cultural considerations in preparing to provide patient education. Some strategies that may be effective in teaching an Hispanic adult with diabetes include providing the patient with written materials in both English and Spanish, providing a one-on-one educational session, and including the family in teaching sessions. Providing culturally appropriate interventions will help to ensure the effectiveness of the teaching provided.

161. B: Clinician. The Iowa Model of Evidence-Based Practice to Promote Quality of Care is one of the evidence-based practice models that view the steps in the evidence-based practice process from the viewpoint of the clinician. The advantage of this viewpoint is that input from the end user is used to determine an area of improving care based on evidence, prioritization based on organizational needs, formulation of a team of key stakeholders, synthesis of evidence with subsequent evidence-based practice recommendations, and evaluation of changes.

162. D: The investigation of methods, variables, and interventions that influence the adoption of evidence-based practices to improve clinical and operational decision making. Translation science is the investigation of methods, variables, and interventions that influence the adoption of evidence-based practices to improve clinical and operation decision making in the healthcare

environment. Analysis of the effectiveness of evidence-based interventions to promote and sustain the adoption of evidence-based practices is included in translation science. The integration of best research evidence, clinical expertise, and patient values to guide clinical care is evidence-based practice. A set of concepts, definitions, relationships, and propositions derived from nursing models or other disciplines that project a purposive systematic view of phenomena is a nursing theory. A theory or group of ideas about how something should be done or thought about is a paradigm.

163. D: Relief, ease, and transcendence. Katharine Kolcaba's theory of comfort is a middle range theory that was developed in the 1990s. Comfort is a desirable outcome of nursing and a product of the art of holistic nursing. In her theory, Kolcaba describes comfort existing in the following 3 forms: relief, ease, and transcendence.

164. B: Avoiding. Interpersonal conflict may be handled by using certain conflict management strategies. There are many different conflict management strategies that have been identified in the literature, including dominating, obliging, avoiding, compromising, and integrating. The type of style used may depend on the situation and the parties involved. In this scenario, the nurse manager used avoidance by not addressing the comments made by the CNS and walking away from the situation. The use of this strategy may have caused the CNS to feel frustrated and powerless, and that the impact of adding this onto her already busy workload was not considered. Compromising may have been a more useful strategy in this scenario. The nurse manager may have offered to pick a better date and time in exchange for the CNS's help with the staff education, or have offered to assist her in lightening her workload by providing additional resources so that she could fit the education into her schedule.

165. C: "I really enjoy working here and with you. I am hoping we can take a look at the way we complete the assignment to make the workload manageable for the both of us." There are many different communication strategies that can be utilized to manage and/or avoid conflict. Using absolute statements like "you always" or "you never" should be avoided. Moderating terms such as "often" or "possibly" are preferred over the use of words like "worst," "most," or "fewest." The use of the word "but" is not recommended as it may elicit defensiveness. The word "and" may be used in place of "but." Using the individual in the definition of the problem is also not recommended.

166. D: Speaking low and slowly, using relaxed body language. Some helpful communication strategies that can be utilized in conflict resolution include the following: the use of open-ended and clarifying questions, focusing on the individual speaking, minimizing distractions, use of kind and caring language, keeping your voice low and speaking slowly, using relaxed body language, leaving individuals out of the definition of the problem, and being objective.

167. B: Patient satisfaction. Patient-centered care involves a partnership among practitioners, patients, and families that is based on viewing the patient as a whole person, effective communication and patient involvement in his or her own care, and consideration of a patient's ability to understand. In addition, patient-centered care takes into consideration a patient's own needs and values. The impact of patient-centered care includes greater patient satisfaction and compliance, lessening of symptoms, and reductions in misdiagnoses due to improved patient communication.

168. C: Emotional intelligence. Emotional intelligence is defined as the ability of a person to recognize, understand, and evaluate one's own emotions as well as the emotions of others to guide their thinking and actions. It is a skill shown to be useful in providing patient-centered care, increasing quality of work and productivity.

169. B: Encouraging behavioral changes. The World Health Organization developed a falls prevention model that provides a comprehensive framework for reducing falls and fall-related injuries in the geriatric population. The 3 pillars of the model include building awareness, identification and assessment of risk factors, and identification and implementation of realistic and effective fall prevention interventions. Encouraging behavioral changes may be considered as an intervention for those patients showing high fall-risk behaviors.

170. A: Late menopause. Osteoporosis is a condition that may lead to falls, as pathologic fractures often precede a fall. Risk factors include increased age, female gender, smoking, low body weight and small stature, family history, white or Asian race, early menopause, excessive alcohol use, physical inactivity, high caffeine intake, and the use of certain medications such as steroids or heparin.

171. D: All of the above. Studies aimed at exploring nurse's awareness, knowledge, and attitude toward evidence-based practice have revealed an overall positive attitude towards adoption and implementation of evidence-based practice. Heavy workloads impacting time often make it difficult for a registered nurse to keep up with current evidence and recommendations. In addition, other barriers such as the inability to understand statistical terminology and evidence-based research may also play a role in a nurse's ability to adopt evidence-based research into clinical practice.

172. D: Nursing theory. Healthcare providers need specific skills and competencies to provide and enhance the quality and safety of patient care. In the 2011 report, *The Future of Nursing: Leading Change, Advancing Health*, the Institute of Medicine recommended that all healthcare providers possess the skills necessary to advance patient care quality and safety. Those skills include patient-centered care, teamwork and collaboration, evidence-based practice, quality improvement, safety, and informatics.

173. B: Personal experience. Evidence-based practice is defined as the integration of best research evidence, clinical expertise, and patient values to guide clinical care. Key components of evidence-based practice include clinical expertise, patient values and preferences, and current research evidence. Research evidence may include qualitative and outcomes research and clinical trials. Clinical expertise may include knowledge gained from practice and inductive reasoning. Patient values may include preferences, concerns, and expectations of their healthcare experience.

174. C: Ask clinical questions using patient scenarios. The next step in the evidence-based practice process would be the assessment of the current practice using patient-specific scenarios to frame the clinical question. The clinical question should be searchable and answerable. Clinical questions should take into consideration the population, intervention or topic of interest, comparison and intervention groups, outcomes, and time.

175. C: Decreased body water. As a person ages there are certain physiologic conditions that have the potential to affect the manner in which drugs are distributed in the body. Increased fat mass, decreased muscle mass, and decreased body water all have the potential to affect drug distribution. Serum albumin decreases with age and rapid reduction in serum albumin may enhance a drug's effects. The risk of toxicity with phenytoin and warfarin is greater in patients with decreased serum albumin levels.

# Practice Test #2

## Practice Questions

1. If the CNS is caring for a patient who has a history of cocaine abuse, for which of the following health problems should the CNS be alert?
    a. memory impairment and respiratory depression
    b. uncontrolled tremors, cardiac dysrhythmias, and impaired cognition
    c. sexual dysfunction, gastric ulcers, and glomerulonephritis
    d. nasal sores and septal perforation and cardiac dysrhythmias

2. According to his son, a 70-year-old man whose wife died 6 months earlier appeared to grieve little and manage well after her death, resuming an active social life, but has become increasingly withdrawn in the past month, eating and sleeping poorly and wandering the house at night. The patient is hospitalized with depression. Which of the following in a priority intervention for the CNS?
    a. Encourage the patient to think about the future.
    b. Encourage the patient to talk about his wife and her death.
    c. Encourage the patient to eat nutritious meals.
    d. Encourage the patient to establish a sleeping schedule.

3. If a patient is on bedrest with myocarditis, the toileting option that the CNS should recommend is
    a. Foley catheter and bedpan.
    b. bedpan.
    c. bedside commode.
    d. bathroom privileges.

4. A 33-year-old woman is hospitalized for treatment of acute pyelonephritis and has been receiving IV fluids and ampicillin plus aminoglycoside for the past 5 days, but the patient's temperature remains elevated and the patient is still in pain and nauseated. The patient should likely be evaluated for
    a. perinephric abscess.
    b. pelvic inflammatory disease.
    c. allergic reaction to drugs.
    d. urinary tract obstruction.

5. A patient who suffered a stroke has persistent dysphagia and cough, and the CNS is concerned that the patient may aspirate. Which of the following referrals is *most appropriate*?
    a. Physical therapist
    b. Occupational therapist
    c. Respiratory therapist
    d. Speech pathologist

6. If a 56-year-old patient is admitted for possible pancreatitis, which of the following laboratory tests are needed on admission in order to apply Ranson's criteria?
   a. WBC, troponin, and calcium
   b. WBC, BUN, calcium, and glucose
   c. WBC, glucose, AST, and LDH
   d. WBC, BUN, AST, and LDH

7. If the CNS works with a population that includes males having sex with males (MSM), the CNS should recommend the HPV vaccination for
   a. MSM ≤ 35 years of age
   b. MSM ≤ 26 years of age
   c. MSM ≤ 21 years of age
   d. MSM ≤ 18 years of age

8. A 28-year-old patient with 3 young children has ovarian cancer and is to be discharged to her home with fentanyl transdermal patches for pain control. When teaching the patient about the use of the patches, the CNS should stress that discarded patches
   a. must be immediately flushed down the toilet.
   b. can be discarded into any waste basket.
   c. should be cut into small pieces before discarding.
   d. can be discarded in any manner because they are harmless.

9. A 76-year-old woman ate *E. coli* (O157:H7)–contaminated vegetables and developed abdominal cramps and non-bloody diarrhea that persisted for 48 hours after which the diarrhea became bloody and has remained so for 4 days. If the patient's condition does not resolve, the patient is at risk of development of
   a. intestinal necrosis.
   b. small bowel obstruction.
   c. intestinal perforation.
   d. hemolytic uremic syndrome.

10. If the CNS is conducting clinical research and intends to select participants who will be able to provide a particular perspective related to the research question, this type of sampling is referred to as
    a. purposeful.
    b. nominated.
    c. convenience.
    d. theoretical.

11. The CNS is leading an ad hoc team that is utilizing failure mode and effects analysis (FMEA) to identify potential failures in the system that may result in increased healthcare-associated infections. Once a list of potential failures is compiled, calculation of the risk priority number (RPN) is based on
    a. objectives and goals.
    b. severity, occurrence, and detection.
    c. inputs, throughputs, and outputs.
    d. analysis, design, and development.

12. Which of the following statements by a patient indicates that the CNS needs to provide education?
    a. "I take all kinds of herbal medicines because I know they're always safe."
    b. "I stopped eating grapefruit because it interacts with so many medications."
    c. "I always try to look up the side effects of medicines I'm taking."
    d. "I take acetaminophen for headache instead of NSAIDs or aspirin."

13. A 49-year-old man has severe chest pain radiating to the left shoulder and arm. Vital signs include BP 152/92 mm Hg, pulse rate of 96 bpm, and respiratory rate of 20 breaths/minute. Oxygen saturation is 94% and temperature is 38°C (100.4°F). The patient is nauseated, and the skin is clammy. ECG shows anterior STEMI. Treatment priority should include
    a. beta-blocker.
    b. ACE inhibitor.
    c. oxygen.
    d. ASA and nitrate.

14. If a 64-year-old female patient has persistent overflow incontinence, the treatment that the CNS should recommend is
    a. urinary diversion.
    b. Foley catheter.
    c. intermittent catheterization.
    d. protective pads.

15. The CNS is working on a unit that has been understaffed. One of the nurses on the unit states that his blood pressure has increased because he dreads coming to work and feels that the organization does not value nurses or care about patients and that nothing will change. The CNS should recognize that the nurse is most at risk for
    a. workplace violence.
    b. burnout.
    c. accidental injury.
    d. negligent patient care.

16. As team leader, the CNS must work collaboratively with a number of team members. When the CNS is delegating a task, the delegation process should begin with
    a. specific timeline for completion of the task.
    b. identification of necessary resources.
    c. identification of priorities.
    d. the task to be delegated and the expected outcomes.

17. The CNS walks by a patient's room and notes that the patient's upper side rails are elevated and the patient's bed is in high position while the patient is unattended. The CNS should lower the bed and
    a. discuss safety issues with staff members.
    b. determine who left the bed in high position.
    c. notify the supervisor.
    d. take no further action.

18. Which of the following is a realistic goal for the CNS to include in the care plan of a patient with diabetes mellitus?
    a. A1c < 5%
    b. A1c < 7%
    c. preprandial glucose of 60 to 100 mg/dL
    d. postprandial glucose of < 120 mg/dL

19. A patient newly diagnosed with tuberculosis is taking isoniazid (INH). Which vitamin should the CNS advise the patient to take prevent peripheral neuropathy?
    a. vitamin C
    b. vitamin A
    c. vitamin B6 (pyridoxine)
    d. vitamin B12 (cobalamin)

20. If the CNS is promoting evidence-based practice and using the PICOT format to pose a clinical question, the CNS would first focus on
    a. personal interests.
    b. philosophy of care.
    c. placement of resources.
    d. patient population.

21. A patient being treated for endocarditis has developed sudden onset of hematuria. The CNS should alert the physician regarding possible
    a. renal embolization
    b. urinary tract infection.
    c. drug reaction.
    d. bladder hemorrhage.

22. A volunteer who is a native speaker of the language of a priority population translated health education program materials for the CNS without being asked. Before utilizing the materials, the CNS should
    a. assume the materials are translated correctly.
    b. verify the translations with a professional translator.
    c. ask English speakers among the priority population to check translation.
    d. assume the materials are translated incorrectly.

23. If the CNS is conducting classes regarding infection control and is developing goals, objectives, strategies, and lesson plans, which of the following would be a *strategy*?
    a. Increase compliance with handwashing standards.
    b. Observe 100% compliance with handwashing.
    c. Place handwashing posters in all nursing units.
    d. Discussion period—The nurse's role in reducing infection.

24. If a patient is undergoing thrombolytic infusion for pulmonary emboli and must have a venipuncture for laboratory tests, manual pressure should be applied to the venipuncture site for at least
    a. 5 minutes.
    b. 10 minutes.
    c. 15 minutes.
    d. 30 minutes.

25. A 70-year-old woman with COPD has experienced an exacerbation after contracting an upper respiratory infection. The patient's oxygen saturation level on admission is 84%. Blood gases are pH 7.29, $PaCO_2$ 52 mm Hg, $PaO_2$ 53 mm Hg, and $HCO_3$ 25 mEq/L. Based on these findings, the acid-base imbalance the patient is experiencing is
   a. respiratory alkalosis.
   b. respiratory acidosis.
   c. metabolic alkalosis.
   d. metabolic acidosis.

26. The CNS works with a group of ethnically diverse staff members, but a number of conflicts have arisen because of different methods of communication and attitudes toward authority. The *best* solution is likely to
   a. initiate a discussion about cultural differences.
   b. issue guidelines regarding effective communication.
   c. ignore the situation and give it time to resolve.
   d. seek outside assistance in conflict resolution.

27. A 27-year-old male patient has had increased thirst and frequency of urination, including nocturia. He has had increased appetite but lost 4 pounds in the previous 2-week period. Laboratory tests show glucose level of 526 mg/dL (29.2 mmol/L), urine positive for glucose and ketones, and blood pH of 7.22. The blood pH is the result of
   a. a normal finding.
   b. increased urinary output.
   c. increased fluid intake.
   d. increased ketone levels in blood.

28. If the CNS needs to interview a patient and the patient is lying supine in bed because of a back injury, the *best* means of ensuring a therapeutic interaction is for the CNS to
   a. stand and talk to the patient.
   b. assist the patient to sit up.
   c. pull up a chair and sit at bedside.
   d. return when the patient is out of bed.

29. A 24-year-old patient was diagnosed with type 1 diabetes mellitus after presenting with a glucose level of 468 mg/dL (26 mmol/L), polyuria, polydipsia, and weight loss. His condition has stabilized since starting insulin injections, and the patient now appears to be able to manage the diabetes with very little insulin. The CNS should suspect that
   a. the patient's insulin needs will increase again.
   b. the patient will no longer need to take insulin.
   c. the patient was misdiagnosed and has type 2 diabetes.
   d. the patient's condition will remain stable at this level.

30. If the CNS is collaborating with the public health department on an initiative to collect data about community needs, the first step should be to define the
   a. methodology.
   b. resources.
   c. needs.
   d. population.

31. A 32-year-old woman reports repeated episodes of palpitation 6 to 10 times daily. The patient has experienced increased irritability, insomnia, heat intolerance, and eye irritation. The patient has lost 5 pounds in the previous month. Vital signs are BP 170/86 mm Hg, pulse rate of 114 bpm, and respiratory rate 20 breaths/minute. Temperature is 37.5°C (99.5°F), and ECG shows atrial fibrillation. Which of the following diagnostic tests are most indicated?
    a. renal function tests
    b. cardiac enzymes
    c. thyroid function tests
    d. liver function tests

32. If a 19-year-old female patient with sickle cell disease experienced an aplastic crisis and has a hemoglobin level of 5.6 g/dL (56 mmol/L), the patient will likely receive transfusions of packed red blood cells until the patient's hemoglobin reaches
    a. 8 g/dL (80 mmol/L).
    b. 10 g/dL (100 mmol/L).
    c. 12 g/dL (120 mmol/L).
    d. 14 g/dL (140 mmol/L).

33. A 46-year-old patient suffered blood loss in a motor vehicle accident. The patient's hemoglobin is 14.1 and hematocrit is 43%, ECG shows slight ST depression, BUN is 28 mg/dL (11.42 mmol/L), creatinine 2 mg/dL (221 micromol/L), ALT 42 IU/L, and AST 49 IU (0.83 microkat/L). These findings most likely represent
    a. hypovolemia and liver ischemia.
    b. normal values.
    c. minor anemia related to blood loss.
    d. acute renal injury.

34. A 78-year-old patient with COPD is hospitalized with acute respiratory distress syndrome (ARDS) and pronounced wheezing, fever (38.6°C [101.5°F]), and cough. Arterial blood gases are pH 7.24, PaO$_2$ 49 mm Hg, and PaCO$_2$ 61 mm Hg. The patient is provided steroids and bronchodilators and is alert and able to follow directions but unable to speak because of dyspnea. Which treatment is *most appropriate* to relieve respiratory distress?
    a. oxygen therapy only
    b. intubation and assist/control (AC) ventilation
    c. intubation and synchronized intermittent mandatory ventilation (SIMV)
    d. non-invasive ventilation (NIV).

35. Which of the following characteristics helps to distinguish an asthma attack from a COPD exacerbation?
    a. Asthma lacks a genetic component.
    b. Most asthma patients are smokers.
    c. Onset of asthma is usually younger than 30 years.
    d. Asthma attacks respond less quickly to treatment.

36. Which of the following clinical signs or symptoms observed by the CNS may indicate that an abdominal aortic aneurysm rupture is imminent?
    a. bounding pulses distal to aneurysm
    b. sudden lumbar pain radiating to the flank and groin
    c. tenderness over area of aneurysm
    d. hypertensive crisis

37. A patient was hit in the head with a hard ball and lost consciousness for a brief period but was then alert and responsive. However, the patient became unstable 2 hours later with severe headache, visual disturbances, nausea and vomiting, and seizures. Which of the following tests should the patient undergo to confirm a diagnosis of epidural hematoma?
    a. MRI
    b. x-ray
    c. CT
    d. cerebral angiograms

38. A patient who was the victim of a violent assault and rape is shaking and crying and appears terrified. Which of the following responses is most therapeutic at the initial encounter with the patient?
    a. "Why are you crying?"
    b. "I can see you are still frightened."
    c. "What can I do to help you?"
    d. "You are safe now."

39. Which of the following teaching strategies is the most efficient approach for a group of 8 patients regarding the need for lifestyle changes required to manage hypertension and heart disease?
    a. discussion
    b. lecture-discussion
    c. role playing
    d. demonstration/Return demonstration

40. The CNS examines a patient's functional ability and notes that the patient's gait is characterized by shuffling of the feet with periodic short, rapid steps while the neck, trunk, and knees are flexed, while the patient leans forward, increasingly walking faster. This CNS should recognize this gait as characteristic of
    a. Parkinson disease.
    b. cerebral palsy.
    c. hemiplegia.
    d. developmental dysplasia of the hip.

41. When conducting a history and physical exam of a patient with dyspnea, the CNS discovers that the patient has smoked 1.5 packs (30) cigarettes daily for at least 15 years. How many pack-years does this represent?
    a. 10
    b. 20
    c. 30
    d. 40

42. A patient with fractured ribs resulted in a left pneumothorax of about 12%. The CNS anticipates that the treatment will include
    a. needle aspiration.
    b. chest tube insertion at left 4th or 5th intercostal space on the midaxillary line.
    c. chest tube insertion at the left 2nd intercostal space on midclavicular line.
    d. supplemental oxygen.

43. A patient with HIV/AIDS and a history of drug abuse has moved home with aging parents who are not supportive. The patient has become quite depressed and requires assistance with ADLs and treatment, frequently misses appointments, and fails to follow treatment regimen, the patient's characteristic is best described as
    a. resilient.
    b. vulnerable.
    c. complex.
    d. stable.

44. If a patient with a suspected brain tumor exhibits lack of coordination, memory loss, and speech difficulties, the most likely tumor location is the
    a. frontal lobe.
    b. temporal lobe.
    c. parietal lobe.
    d. occipital lobe.

45. A patient is experiencing an acute episode of asthma and is anxious, sitting in tripod position with audible wheezing resulting from upper airway obstruction. The patient's peak flow is 65% of normal and oxygen saturation is 92%. The initial rescue protocol should begin with
    a. albuterol.
    b. prednisone or methylprednisolone.
    c. antihistamine, such as diphenhydramine.
    d. theophylline.

46. If a patient with acute pericarditis has severe sternal pain radiating to the neck and increasing on inspiration, the CNS should advise the patient to
    a. lie flat in supine position.
    b. lie in left lateral Sims position.
    c. sit in semi-Fowler's position.
    d. sit up and lean forward.

47. A 60-year-old African American patient presented with BMI of 32 kg/m$^2$, hemoglobin A1c level of 7.1, fasting serum glucose of 152 mg/dL (8.4 mmol/L), triglyceride level of 168, and HDL 24 mg/dL. The patient is diagnosed with insulin resistance and diabetes mellitus, type 2. Which of the following is usually the drug of choice to initiate therapy?
    a. Sulfonylureas, such as glimepiride.
    b. Biguanide, such as metformin.
    c. Meglitinide, such as repaglinide.
    d. Alpha-glucosidase inhibitor, such as acarbose.

48. According to the WHO three-step ladder approach to pain management, if a patient's abdominal pain associated with pancreatic cancer varies from 4 to 8 on the pain scale, pain control should be initiated at
    a. step 1.
    b. step 2.
    c. step 3.
    d. whichever step is appropriate at the time of initiation.

49. A patient under end-of-life hospice care for stage 4 multiple myeloma has developed severe skeletal pain and is scheduled to undergo radiation therapy to reduce discomfort. How will this treatment affect hospice care?
   a. Hospice care must be discontinued.
   b. Hospice care is put on hold until treatment finished and then resumed.
   c. Hospice care will continue without interruption.
   d. Hospice care may be continued if preauthorization is received.

50. Following lunch at a restaurant, a 72-year-old female experiences a sudden episode of loss of vision in the right eye. At the same time, the patient feels dizzy and weak, and her speech is slightly garbled, but the symptoms clear within 15 to 20 minutes. The most likely diagnosis is
   a. transient ischemic episode (TIE).
   b. stroke.
   c. allergic reaction.
   d. panic attack.

51. A patient being treated for cardiogenic shock after an acute myocardial infarction has an intra-aortic balloon pump (IABP) in place, and the radiology technician has arrived in the unit to take a portable chest x-ray in order to evaluate the degree of pulmonary edema. When the CNS observes the technician preparing to sit the patient upright in order to place the cassette film holder behind the patient's back, the CNS should
   a. assist the technician.
   b. remind the patient to flex the knees.
   c. immediately stop the technician.
   d. monitor the patient's VS during the procedure.

52. If a patient is admitted to the ED for an ischemic stroke, the most essential laboratory tests prior to thrombolysis are
   a. complete blood cell count.
   b. renal function tests.
   c. serum glucose and coagulation studies.
   d. liver function tests.

53. If a patient involved in a motor vehicle accident has bruising over the area of the mastoid process (Battle's sign) as well as bilateral "raccoon eyes" (swollen, ecchymotic), the injury consistent with the clinical signs is
   a. frontal skull fracture.
   b. basilar skull fracture.
   c. temporoparietal skull fracture.
   d. occipital skull fracture.

54. Which of the following patients is most at risk of development of a chronic subdural hematoma 3 to 4 weeks after initial injury?
   a. 18-year-old patient who developed a concussion from a football injury
   b. 28-year old patient who struck her head on a water ski
   c. 46-year-old patient who had lacerations of the forehead in a motor vehicle accident
   d. 78-year-old patient who fell and hit the head on the floor but experienced only a slight headache

55. The AVPU assessment is done after head injury to determine the patient's
    a. level of consciousness.
    b. intracranial pressure.
    c. degree of brain injury.
    d. motor abilities.

56. The medical-surgical unit has experienced an outbreak of *Clostridium difficile* infections involving 10 patients over a 2-week period. In order to reduce further transmission of the infection, the CNS is working with staff members and should concentrate efforts on
    a. contact precautions/hand hygiene.
    b. antibiotic stewardship.
    c. testing patient stool specimens.
    d. limiting patient contacts.

57. A patient was stung by a bee and has pain and itching around the site of the bee sting with erythema and edema extending about 8 cm diameter around the site. The patient has no systemic manifestations. What initial medication is indicated in addition to removal of the stinger and application of an ice pack?
    a. epinephrine
    b. antihistamine, such as diphenhydramine (Benadryl)
    c. corticosteroid, such as prednisone
    d. no medication is indicated

58. Using the Rule of 9s to estimate the body surface area (BSA) of a patient who experienced burns from toxic chemicals, if the patient has burns covering the chest (but not the abdomen) and the anterior surface of the left arm, the BSA with burns is approximately
    a. 27%.
    b. 18%.
    c. 13.5%.
    d. 9%.

59. A patient involved in a motor vehicle accident had multiple injuries, including fractured ribs, an unstable posterior ring pelvic fracture, and blunt trauma to the liver. The patient required transfusions for blood loss, and the pelvic fracture was stabilized by external fixation. The liver trauma was treated with nonoperative management. During the recovery period, the patient is most at risk of
    a. hemorrhage.
    b. infection.
    c. disseminated intravascular coagulopathy (DIC).
    d. deep vein thrombosis (DVT).

60. A patient taking sertraline for depression noted a decrease in urinary output over a 1-month period. Serum sodium level was 120 mEq/L (120 mmol/L). The patient exhibited mild confusion, anorexia, and nausea, and was diagnosed with SIADH. Sertraline, which is associated with hyponatremia, was discontinued and patient's sodium levels monitored. What first-line intervention does the CNS expect?
    a. fluid limitation
    b. IV sodium
    c. oral sodium
    d. loop diuretic

61. An older patient tells the CNS that she is very concerned that her end-of-life care provides comfort and avoids unnecessary interventions. Which of the following is the *best* recommendation for the patient?
    a. power of attorney
    b. advance directive
    c. DNR request form
    d. will

62. If a patient is admitted to the hospital with a diagnosis of left ventricular heart failure, which of the following clinical indications does the CNS expect?
    a. abdominal distention
    b. ankle edema
    c. weight gain
    d. dyspnea and cough

63. A patient's cardiac monitor shows the following heart pattern:

    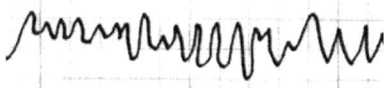

    Based on this ECG recording, what emergent treatment should the CNS anticipate?
    a. observation only
    b. beta-blocker
    c. defibrillation
    d. amiodarone

64. A patient with end-stage renal disease develops a hypertensive crisis with BP 182/108 mm Hg, pulse rate of 104 bpm, respiratory rate of 18 breaths/minute, and oxygen saturation 98%. The patient is anxious and complains of headache, but there is no indication of organ damage. The patient is administered labetalol by infusion. How much reduction in BP should the CNS expect over the first 6 hours after treatment is initiated?
    a. 10%
    b. 33%
    c. 66%
    d. 100%

65. A patient is recovering from CABG and is ambulating in the hallway with a wireless cardiac monitor when an alarm sounds indicating that the patient is experiencing supraventricular tachycardia with a pulse rate of 162 bpm. Which of the following interventions should take priority?
    a. Take the patient's BP.
    b. Walk the patient back to the bed.
    c. Notify the physician.
    d. Assist the patient to sit down.

66. If a post-anesthesia patient just awakening following removal of the intubation tube begins to cough and aspiration of gastric fluids is suspected, the CNS should immediately
   a. Lower the patient's head and turn the patient to the side.
   b. Do endotracheal suctioning.
   c. Increase oxygen to 6 L per mask.
   d. Sit the patient upright and encourage deep breathing.

67. A patient with heart failure has developed pulmonary edema and has audible wheeze with rales and rhonchi present throughout the lung fields. The patient is quite anxious. The patient is initially treated with oxygen at 15 L per non-rebreather mask, furosemide 60 mg IV, as well as nitroglycerine and nitroprusside to increase peripheral vasodilation and morphine to reduce anxiety. The initial goal of therapy should be to maintain $PaO_2$ above
   a. 40 mm Hg.
   b. 60 mm Hg.
   c. 70 mm Hg.
   d. 80 mm Hg.

68. If a 64-year-old African American male patient with diabetes has BP readings that average about 154/96 mm Hg, the first-line pharmacologic therapy that the CNS should advise is
   a. thiazide diuretic or calcium channel blocker.
   b. ACE inhibitor and ARB.
   c. thiazide diuretic or ARB.
   d. loop diuretic.

69. If a 56-year-old patient experienced blunt thoracic trauma during a motor vehicle accident at 20 mph, the *most appropriate* initial diagnostic tool to assess for cardiac trauma is a(n)
   a. chest x-ray.
   b. ECG.
   c. echocardiogram.
   d. coronary angiogram.

70. Following cardiac surgery for repair of aortic valve, the patient has acute chest pain and shortness of breath, relieved by sitting up and learning forward. The patient is pale, diaphoretic, and hypotensive, and peripheral pulses are rapid and weak with paradoxical pulse noted and narrow pulse pressure. The CNS should prepare the patient for emergent
   a. thrombolysis.
   b. ECG.
   c. pericardiocentesis.
   d. angiograms.

71. Which of the following interactions between the CNS and a patient of a different ethnic and cultural backgrounds indicates the CNS's cultural responsiveness?
   a. The CNS discusses the purpose and meaning of the medical regimen.
   b. The CNS informs the patient of the critical nature of medical adherence.
   c. The CNS tells the patient that cultural health practices are inadequate.
   d. The CNS sends someone of the same ethnic/cultural background to speak with the patient.

72. If a patient is taking atorvastatin for dyslipidemia, which of the following medications may the CNS recommend for its additive effect to reduce the risk of cardiac mortality resulting from dyslipidemia?
   a. bile acid sequestrant
   b. cholesterol absorption inhibitor
   c. fibrate
   d. MTP inhibitor

73. A patient with acute respiratory failure (ARF) is intubated and receiving mechanical ventilation. Which of the following steps are important to prevent ventilator-associated pneumonia (VAP)?
   a. Keep head of bed at 60 to 90 degrees.
   b. Brush teeth daily with hydrogen peroxide.
   c. Maintain sedation at the same level.
   d. DVT prophylaxis

74. If a patient has increasing intracranial pressure (ICP), the aim of treatment is to maintain the ICP at
   a. 20 to 25 mm Hg.
   b. < 20 mm Hg.
   c. 10 to 15 mm Hg.
   d. 5 to 10 mm Hg.

75. A patient with multiple anterior and posterior coronary artery obstructions is scheduled for an on-pump coronary artery bypass graft (CABG) but asks the nurse why she was not a candidate for the minimally invasive direct CABG. The *most appropriate* response is to tell the patient that minimally invasive direct CABG
   a. requires special equipment and training that is not available at this site.
   b. is used only for one-vessel disease in anterior (front) portions of the coronary arteries.
   c. is associated with more complications than on-pump CABG.
   d. is not covered by most insurance companies or Medicare.

76. A patient in minor alcohol withdrawal is prescribed chlordiazepoxide. The purpose of this benzodiazepine is to
   a. prevent delirium and seizures.
   b. prevent Wernicke encephalopathy.
   c. treat psychosis.
   d. treat active seizures.

77. If a Navajo patient tells the CNS that he has "ghost sickness," the *most appropriate* response is
   a. "There is no such disease."
   b. "What do you mean?"
   c. "Is that a common name for a real illness?"
   d. "How does ghost sickness make you feel?"

78. If a patient has suspected heart failure, which of the following tests should the CNS expect will show the severity of the heart failure?
   a. C-reactive protein (CRP)
   b. homocysteine
   c. ischemia-modified albumin (IMA)
   d. B-type natriuretic peptide (BNP)

79. A patient with hypertrophic cardiomyopathy has been prescribed propranolol. The CNS should inform the patient and family members that patients taking the drug are at risk of
    a. tachycardia.
    b. depression.
    c. hypertension.
    d. anorexia.

80. The CNS is examining a patient with circulatory impairment of the lower extremities. Which of the following should the CNS recognize as an indication of arterial insufficiency?
    a. brownish discoloration around ankles
    b. moderate to severe edema
    c. pedal pulse present
    d. rubor on dependency and pallor on elevation

81. If a 50-year-old female patient has symptoms consistent with mitral stenosis, when completing the history and physical exam, the CNS should ask specifically about a history of
    a. rheumatic fever.
    b. cardiac trauma.
    c. myocardial infarction.
    d. Marfan syndrome.

82. If the CNS is using the BVMGR (beliefs, values, meanings, goals, and relationships) rubric for implementing spiritual care, these aspects apply to the
    a. the CNS.
    b. the culture.
    c. the patient.
    d. the organization.

83. When the CNS is assisting a physician with synchronized cardioversion for a patient in atrial fibrillation, before the physician places the paddles, the CNS should check the machine to ensure it is properly sensing
    a. P waves.
    b. Q waves.
    c. R waves.
    d. ST waves.

84. A 68-year-old man in good health has sudden onset of severe weakness, chest pain, dyspnea, cough, and low-grade fever of 38°C (100.4°F). The patient's systolic BP is palpable at 52 mm Hg, pulse is 128 bpm, respiratory rate of 38 breaths/minute, and oxygen saturation 81% on room air. Which of the following tests may provide the *best* information to rule out pulmonary embolism?
    a. D-dimer assay
    b. arterial blood gases
    c. CBC
    d. PTT

85. If the Richmond Agitation and Sedation Scale (RASS) is used to help titrate sedation for a patient with acute lung injury (ALI) who is intubated and receiving mechanical ventilation, the CNS should ensure that the RASS score is maintained at
    a. -1 to -2.
    b. -3 to -4.
    c. +1 to +2.
    d. +3 to +4.

86. A 42-year-old woman had a laparoscopic cholecystectomy and did well initially, but in the previous 24 hours, the patient has developed severe nausea and vomiting, unrelieved with ondansetron (Zofran). The patient exhibits increasing confusion and experiences a tonic-clonic seizure. The patient's electrolytes show potassium 4 mEq/L (4 mmol/L) and sodium 123 mEq/L (123 mmol/L). If the CNS is to administer 100 mL of 3% NaCl over 10 minutes and to repeat up to 3 times as needed to increase the sodium level, the initial goal for increase in the first hour to prevent brain herniation is
    a. 1 to 3 mEq/L (1 to 3 mmol/L).
    b. 4 to 6 mEq/L (4 to 6 mmol/L).
    c. 7 to 8 mEq/L (7 to 8 mmol/L)
    d. 9 to 10 mEq/L (9 to 10 mmol/L).

87. The CNS is evaluating a patient with a history of aortic insufficiency. For which of the following complications should the CNS plan to assess the patient?
    a. atrial fibrillation
    b. heart block
    c. right-sided heart failure
    d. left-sided heart failure

88. Which of the following increases the risk of aspiration for a patient receiving NG feedings?
    a. head elevated at 45 degree
    b. continuous feeding
    c. young age
    d. history of diabetes mellitus

89. Which of the following types of aspirations does the CNS expect to produce the most severe pulmonary damage?
    a. acid liquid (such as liquid gastric contents)
    b. nonacid liquid (such as water)
    c. acid food particles (such as partially digested gastric contents)
    d. nonacid food particles (such as chewed bread)

90. If the CNS is educating a patient with obstructive sleep apnea, and the patient is to utilize a BiPAP machine after discharge, the CNS should stress that the patient
    a. must use the BiPAP machine whenever sleeping.
    b. focus on improving diet.
    c. may not need the BiPAP machine during an afternoon nap.
    d. should do deep breathing and coughing exercises.

91. A patient with pulmonary arterial hypertension (WHO II) has started treatment with combination therapy that initially includes ambrisentan 5 mg (Letairis) and tadalafil 20 mg

(Adcirca) as well as supplementary oxygen for exertion. When educating the patient about disease management, the CNS should tell the patient to be especially alert for signs of
   a. unusual bleeding.
   b. peripheral edema.
   c. headache.
   d. dizziness.

92. An HIV-positive 42-year-old man has developed cytomegalovirus pneumonia. A priority intervention should include
   a. supportive care only.
   b. cephalosporin and CMV immune globulin (CMV-IG).
   c. ganciclovir (Cytovene) and CMV immune globulin (CMV-IG).
   d. Valganciclovir (Valcyte) and corticosteroid.

93. If a patient is diagnosed with tuberculosis and must take antituberculosis drugs, for which of the following may the CNS recommend directly observed therapy (DOT)?
   a. Patient has comorbidity with diabetes mellitus.
   b. Patient states he dislikes following treatment regimen.
   c. Patient is low income and lives in Section 8 housing.
   d. Patient is taking methadone for heroin addiction.

94. Adult patients with cystic fibrosis are especially at risk of which type of hospital-acquired pneumonia?
   a. *Staphylococcus aureus* pneumonia
   b. cytomegalovirus (CMV) pneumonia
   c. *Candida* pneumonia
   d. *Pseudomonas aeruginosa* pneumonia

95. If a patient with latex allergy is inadvertently exposed to latex and develops severe anaphylaxis with difficulty breathing, the priority intervention is to establish an airway and administer
   a. oxygen.
   b. epinephrine.
   c. corticosteroid.
   d. albuterol inhaler.

96. If a patient who suffered blunt thoracic trauma exhibits paradoxical movement of the chest during inspiration and expiration with tenderness and crepitation noted on palpation, which of the following tests may provide the *best* diagnostic information?
   a. MRI
   b. MSCT scan and arterial blood gases
   c. chest x-ray
   d. pulmonary function tests

97. A patient who has had a "sore throat and cough" for the previous 5 days comes to the ED with muffled voice and respiratory distress. The patient appears feverish and cyanotic and is sitting in tripod position with the mouth open and tongue out, drooling and leaning forward. Heart rate is 112. The priority intervention should be
    a. establishing an airway.
    b. taking a chest x-ray.
    c. completing a physical exam.
    d. measuring arterial blood gases.

98. If a patient is brought to the ED with a Glasgow Coma Scale score of 12, the CNS expects the patient to be
    a. alert and responsive with no obvious deficits.
    b. completely nonresponsive.
    c. exhibiting decorticate posturing with painful stimuli.
    d. confused but able to follow simple directions.

99. Following craniotomy for removal of a basilar meningioma, a 32-year-old patient experiences increasing thirst and urination. The patient's fasting glucose level is 90 mg/dL (5 mmol/L), CBC is within normal limits, and metabolic panel shows sodium level of 152 mEq/L (152 mmol/L). The urine specific gravity is 1.001. Which of the following tests will provide the *best* diagnostic information?
    a. renal function tests
    b. liver function tests
    c. serum and urine osmolality
    d. renal ultrasound

100. A patient underwent a right pneumonectomy because of malignant lesions. Six days after surgery, the patient exhibits increasing dyspnea and fever and begins to cough up serosanguineous sputum. Chest x-ray shows sudden increased fluid level in the right pleural space. Which of the following complications does the CNS suspect?
    a. acute respiratory failure
    b. hemorrhage
    c. bronchopleural fistula
    d. pulmonary edema

101. According to the Star Model of systems thinking, if the CNS makes a change in one area of nursing care within an organization, the CNS should expect that this will
    a. necessitate a change in another area.
    b. result in discord within the organization.
    c. have little effect on the organization as a whole.
    d. result in positive or negative outcomes.

102. If the CNS feels that the organization is not receptive to change and wants to use a systems approach to facilitating change, the first step is to
    a. describe behavior patterns.
    b. establish cause and effect relationships.
    c. define the issue.
    d. define patterns of performance.

103. If the CNS needs to delegate a task to an LVN/LPN but is unsure how the nurse performs because the CNS has not worked with this LVN/LPN before, the *best* initial approach is to
    a. assign the task and try to observe the LVN/LPN.
    b. ask the LVN/LPN how he or she would go about doing the task.
    c. ask the opinion of nurses who have worked with the LVN/LPN.
    d. outline specific steps to carrying out the task.

104. If the CNS notes that staffing patterns do not always match workload, the first step to a solution is to
    a. complain to management.
    b. organize staff members to demand changes.
    c. determine how staffing decisions are made.
    d. prepare a list of potential changes.

105. The CNS notes that one nursing team member often avoids taking care of older patients and sometimes makes disparaging remarks about them. The *most* appropriate response is for the CNS to
    a. advise the nurse that ageism is inappropriate.
    b. discuss attitudes toward aging with the nurse.
    c. file a complaint against the nurse.
    d. avoid assigning the nurse to older patients.

106. According to the Payne-Martin classification system for skin tears, an example of a category II skin tear is
    a. scant tissue loss: partial thickness injury and ≤ 25% of epidermal flap lost.
    b. linear: full-thickness wound in wrinkle or furrow with epidermis and dermis pulled apart.
    c. flap: partial thickness wound with a flap that can cover wound with ≤ 1 mm of dermis exposed.
    d. complete partial thickness injury with loss of epidermal flap.

107. The CNS must irrigate an open wound with normal saline as part of routine dressing changes. During irrigation, the psi of the irrigant should be no greater than
    a. 4.5 psi.
    b. 8 psi.
    c. 15 psi.
    d. 20 psi.

108. An 80-year-old patient with a history of intraabdominal surgery and diverticulosis has simple incomplete small bowel obstruction (without compromised blood flow) and has had nausea and vomiting for 2 days. Which of the following initial interventions are most indicated?
    a. immediate surgical repair
    b. NG decompression and IV fluids
    c. NG decompression and antibiotic therapy
    d. NG decompression only

109. If the CNS observes unlicensed assistive personnel (UAP) massaging the reddened heels of an immobile patient, the CNS should
   a. file a complaint about the UAP's lack of competence.
   b. compliment the UAP for providing good preventive care.
   c. take no action as this is part of routine care.
   d. explain how massaging reddened tissue may cause tissue damage.

110. A patient's friend is visiting and expresses concern about the patient and asks for an update on the patient's prognosis. The CNS should
   a. provide a general update about the patient without going into detail.
   b. tell the visitor it is not appropriate to ask for information about the patient.
   c. tell the visitor the CNS cannot discuss the patient's condition.
   d. deny knowledge of the patient's prognosis.

111. If a patient has suspected kidney disease, the test that will provide the *best* information about the renal function and the glomerular filtration rate is the
   a. BUN.
   b. serum creatinine.
   c. urinalysis.
   d. creatinine clearance rate.

112. According to systems theory (Bertalanffy), the 5 elements of a system include (1) input, (2) throughput, (3) output, (4) evaluation, and (5)
   a. improvement.
   b. organization.
   c. chaos.
   d. feedback.

113. An 18-year-old patient became angry at her parents and ingested 10,000 mg of extra-strength acetaminophen and was found by her mother 12 hours later. The patient was pale, nauseated, and diaphoretic but had not vomited. The CNS should recognize that the patient is at risk of
   a. renal failure.
   b. liver failure.
   c. intestinal obstruction.
   d. GI bleeding.

114. The hospital administration has collected patient surveys to determine the needs that patients feel are most important. The next step in the quality improvement process should be to
   a. collect data regarding current status of these needs.
   b. determine measurable outcomes.
   c. develop a plan.
   d. assemble a multidisciplinary team.

115. As part of clinical inquiry, the CNS is researching evidence-based practice. Which of the following is a free abstract database that does not require subscription and has many links to publisher's websites?
   a. EMBASE
   b. EBSCO
   c. PubMed
   d. OVID

116. If the CNS is newly hired at a healthcare organization and believes that there is a need for improvement, the first thing the CNS should assess is the
   a. workplace culture.
   b. available resources.
   c. knowledge base of staff.
   d. administrative support.

117. The CNS is encouraging team members to use the STAR approach to patient safety. The CNS explains that the STAR approach begins by
   a. safeguarding patients.
   b. stopping to concentrate on tasks.
   c. securing needed equipment/tools.
   d. selecting appropriate tasks.

118. The CNS is concerned that a number of patients have fallen and has convinced the administration to purchase additional lift equipment and assistive devices. The CNS's next step should be to
   a. post memos stating a zero tolerance for patient falls.
   b. advise the staff members to use the equipment.
   c. develop safety protocols for lifting/handling patients.
   d. post directions for use of lift equipment and assistive devices.

119. If the CNS notes that a patient's BP has fallen precipitously and pulse rate has increased, but he or she fails to inform the patient's physician and the patient suffers permanent injury as a result, the element of malpractice that applies to the CNS is
   a. causation.
   b. foreseeability.
   c. breach of the duty owed.
   d. duty owed to the patient.

120. Which of the following minors may give valid informed consent?
   a. a 17-year-old wanting a rhinoplasty for cosmetic purposes
   b. a 14-year-old giving consent for transfusions against parents' wishes
   c. a 15-year-old male who needs surgery for a fractured femur
   d. a 16-year-old married female

121. If 2 members of the CNS's team have become embroiled in a conflict, which of the follow strategies is an example of the defensive mode of conflict management?
   a. Assign the 2 members to different schedules.
   b. Help the 2 members to arrive at a compromise.
   c. Try to help the 2 members reach a consensus agreement.
   d. Model effective conflict management.

122. If the CNS discovers that a patient faces various problems in returning home after discharge, including lack of adequate income and impaired ability to prepare food, and refers the patient to a social worker for assistance, the type of power that the CNS is exhibiting is
    a. transformational power.
    b. advocacy power.
    c. affirmative power.
    d. integrative power.

123. Generally, the cultural context of patients from which of the following countries would be considered *low* context, that is the meaning comes explicitly from spoken or written words?
    a. Russia
    b. China
    c. Japan
    d. Mexico

124. When working with a diverse group of staff members, the CNS should recognize that the generational group that is most likely to look at duty in terms of personal needs, enjoy teamwork, and expect positive feedback is
    a. Silent Generation.
    b. Baby Boomers.
    c. Generation X.
    d. Millennials.

125. Considering the elements of a system and how it relates to health care, nursing services provided by the CNS would be considered part of
    a. inputs.
    b. throughputs.
    c. outputs.
    d. feedback.

126. If the CNS is in a management position and is basing management strategies on the contingency theory, the leadership style that the CNS would utilize would be
    a. dependent on the situation.
    b. the same under all circumstances.
    c. determined by consensus.
    d. dictated by administration.

127. The CNS has instituted staff rounding with a goal of meeting with each staff member at least once weekly. The purpose of staff rounding is to
    a. update staff members on changes and/or needs.
    b. discuss the staff member's performance issues.
    c. improve communication and support staff members' needs.
    d. eliminate small problems before they become large.

128. If the CNS wants to initiate a process of change in an organization, the CNS must realize that the first essential element of the change is the
    a. decision to bring about change.
    b. understanding the process of change.
    c. taking actions that lead to change.
    d. belief in the possibility of change.

129. When reviewing staffing needs, the CNS finds that staff members' time is most impacted by answering patients' call lights and responding to their needs. Which of the following strategies is likely to be most effective for time saving?
    a. rounding on patients hourly
    b. grouping patients by severity
    c. reminding patients to use the call light only for medical needs
    d. assigning one staff member to answer call lights

130. If an organization has instituted Individualized Patient Care and one of the patients tells the CNS that his idea of excellent care is "to be left in peace and quiet," the CNS should
    a. tell staff members to leave the patient undisturbed.
    b. limit visitors to brief visits only.
    c. clarify what the patient means.
    d. assume the patient is being sarcastic.

131. If a patient is diagnosed with a non–Q-wave myocardial infarction, which of the following characteristics should the CNS anticipate?
    a. abnormal Q waves are evident on ECG
    b. reperfusion will occur spontaneously
    c. infarction will result in necrosis
    d. that the MI is transmural

132. A patient with immune thrombocytopenic purpura (ITP) has a platelet count of $70,000/mm^3$ and is scheduled for a breast biopsy. The CNS notifies the surgeon about the level and should expect the biopsy
    a. to be cancelled because of the low platelet count.
    b. to be carried out after administration of a platelet transfusion.
    c. to be carried out after administration of prednisone.
    d. to be carried out without further treatment.

133. A patient who developed polyarthralgia was recently diagnosed with systemic lupus erythematosus. When educating the patient about lifestyle changes, the CNS should plan to include
    a. dietary modifications.
    b. weight loss and exercise regimens.
    c. energy conservation and skin protection.
    d. bowel care regimens.

134. The CNS should advise a patient who has had a gastrectomy to be monitored routinely for
    a. diabetes mellitus.
    b. anemia.
    c. hypertension.
    d. heart disease.

135. The CNS has taught a patient's spouse to change the patient's dressing and to understand signs of both healing and infection. The *best* method to ensure that the patient's spouse is able to carry out the dressing change and monitor the wound is to ask for a
    a. written test.
    b. verbal description of the procedure.
    c. return demonstration.
    d. follow-up wound assessment.

136. An 18-year-old football player experienced blunt trauma to his left lower leg during a tackle. The patient was able to walk initially with no difficulty. The patient comes to the hospital about an hour later with severe pain and tightness in the lower leg as well as a sensation of burning. The lower leg is edematous and skin taut, although distal pulse is palpable and capillary refill time is within normal limits. The priority intervention should be to
    a. measure compartment pressure.
    b. take an x-ray of the leg.
    c. take CT of the leg.
    d. apply ice packs and elevate the leg.

137. A 32-year-old patient suffered carbon monoxide (CO) toxicity and is receiving 100% oxygen per nonrebreather mask. The patient should be maintained on 100% oxygen therapy until asymptomatic and the hemoglobin CO level falls to below
    a. 20%.
    b. 10%.
    c. 5%.
    d. 2%.

138. An 80-year-old female patient who developed a urinary tract infection now has a temperature of 39°C (102.2°F), pulse of 108 bpm, respiratory rate of 26 breaths/minute, and white blood cell count of 15,000 with 12% bands. Blood cultures are pending. The CNS would classify the patient's stage of infection as
    a. systemic inflammatory response syndrome (SIRS).
    b. severe sepsis.
    c. septic shock.
    d. sepsis.

139. If a 73-year-old patient is admitted from a residential care facility with a coccygeal pressure ulcer that is 6 cm by 4 cm and extends to the muscle and is partially covered with black necrotic tissue, the CNS would classify the pressure ulcer with NPUAP staging as
    a. stage 1.
    b. stage 2
    c. stage 3
    d. stage 4

140. A patient involved in a motorcycle accident fractured the right tibia and fibula and has a new plaster cast that is still damp. The patient says that the cast feels "hot." The CNS should understand that this likely indicates
    a. infection.
    b. bleeding.
    c. circulatory impairment.
    d. normal sensation.

141. The CNS intends to implement a new procedure in the delivery of patient care, understanding that the biggest threat to implementation of change is usually
   a. staff resistance.
   b. lack of adequate preparation.
   c. poor change design.
   d. insufficient supporting data.

142. The stages of team development include (1) forming, (2) storming, (3) norming, (4)_____, and (5) mourning. The fourth stage is
   a. producing.
   b. completing.
   c. accepting.
   d. performing.

143. Which of the following countertransference reactions is the CNS exhibiting if the CNS comes to work early to see a patient who reminds her of her mother, brings the patient small gifts, and is judgmental about the patient's family members' actions?
   a. rescue
   b. misuse of honesty
   c. over-involvement
   d. over-identification

144. A patient with osteomyelitis has not responded adequately to IV antibiotics and is to continue with oral ciprofloxacin after discharge. The patient asks the CNS how progress toward healing will be monitored. The CNS should advise the patient that osteomyelitis is usually monitored with
   a. bone x-rays.
   b. CBC and bone biopsy.
   c. bone biopsy and erythrocyte sedimentation rate (ESR).
   d. bone scans/MRI and ESR.

145. A patient has a temporary external transcutaneous pacemaker in place for bradycardia. After the CNS has adjusted the pacemaker rate setting and identified the pacing threshold, the output setting should be set at
   a. equal to the measured threshold.
   b. 2 to 3 times the measured threshold.
   c. 3 to 4 times the measured threshold.
   d. 4 to 5 times the measured threshold.

146. The CNS is caring for a patient with kidney failure. The patient's GFR has been falling and is 28 ml/min/1.73 m³. At what GFR should the CNS expect that the patient will need to begin renal replacement therapy?
   a. < 30 mL/min/1.73 m2
   b. < 25 mL/min/1.73 m2
   c. < 20 mL/min/1.73 m2
   d. < 15 mL/min/1.73 m2

147. A patient with a history of aggression begins swearing and pacing back and forth, shouting, "You can't make me stay here!" The *best initial* response from the CNS is to
   a. speak calmly and quietly to the patient.
   b. tell the patient this behavior is inappropriate.
   c. leave the room.
   d. call security to restrain the patient.

148.

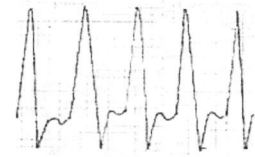

If the CNS is monitoring the waveform during insertion of a pulmonary artery catheter and observes this waveform, the CNS should recognize it as the
   a. right atrial waveform.
   b. right ventricular waveform.
   c. pulmonary arterial waveform.
   d. pulmonary artery occlusion (wedge) waveform.

149. A patient who reports having the "flu" with 3 days of nausea, vomiting, diarrhea with watery stools, and inability to eat or drink anything excepts sips of ginger ale has vital signs of BP 106/82 mm Hg, pulse rate of 90 bpm, and respiratory rate of 24 breaths/minute. Urine specific gravity is 1.036 and serum sodium is 152 mEq/L (152 mmol/L). Serum potassium is 3.1 mEq/L. The CNS should note that the patient's priority treatment is for
   a. hypokalemia only.
   b. deficient fluid volume only.
   c. hyponatremia and hypokalemia.
   d. deficient fluid volume and hypokalemia.

150. A patient with weakness and ascending paralysis reports that he began experiencing symptoms, including tingling and numbness in the lower extremities, a few days before hospitalization. The peripheral reflexes are absent, and the patient is increasingly dyspneic. The patient is diagnosed with Guillain-Barré syndrome and placed on mechanical ventilation. A priority intervention would be
   a. antibiotic therapy.
   b. antiviral therapy.
   c. high-dose immunoglobulin.
   d. corticosteroids.

151. The CNS overhears another nurse complaining that an adult female Hmong patient is subservient and dependent because she allows her father to make decisions about her health care and that the nurse tried without success to convince the patient to make her own decisions. This type of intervention would *best* be described as
   a. ethnocentrism.
   b. cultural imposition.
   c. stereotyping.
   d. cultural competence.

152. When the CNS is assessing a patient with neurological injury, which of the following indicates an upper motor neuron lesion?
   a. muscle spasticity
   b. muscle flaccidity
   c. muscle atrophy
   d. absent reflexes

153. A patient who experienced tonic-clonic seizures is newly diagnosed with epilepsy and has started on anti-seizure medication. When the CNS is educating the patient about the disease, the most important advice is to
   a. avoid all exercise.
   b. tell all family, friends, and associates about the diagnosis.
   c. follow a healthy lifestyle.
   d. never stop taking the medication abruptly.

154. If the CNS is working the night shift and finds it increasingly difficult to stay awake during the night, the *best* way to ensure the CNS is alert during the night is to
   a. sleep immediately after the end of the night shift.
   b. sleep immediately before beginning the night shift.
   c. take short naps during break time.
   d. drink highly caffeinated liquids.

155. If a 25-year-old patient's BMI is 17.5 and the albumin level is normal at 3.8 g/dL (38 g/L) (normal value 3.5 to 5.5 g/dL or 35 to 55 g/L) and prealbumin shows moderate deficiency of 6 mg/dL (60 mg/L) (normal 16 to 40 mg/dL or 160 to 400 mg/L), these findings suggest
   a. long-term protein malnutrition.
   b. short-term protein malnutrition.
   c. adequate protein but inadequate calories.
   d. adequate calories but inadequate protein.

156. If a patient with acute appendicitis awaiting surgery has pain despite analgesia, a non-analgesic measure that may help to alleviate discomfort is
   a. bending the right knee.
   b. turning onto the left side.
   c. lying in flat, supine position.
   d. applying a heating pad to the abdomen.

157. In evaluating research as part of the development of evidence-based practice guidelines, the four evaluative/trustworthiness criteria are (1) credibility, (2) dependability, (3) transferability, and (4)
   a. controllability.
   b. applicability.
   c. accountability.
   d. confirmability.

158. A patient who works in a daycare center and handles food is diagnosed with hepatitis A after developing flu-like symptoms. How long prior to onset of symptoms was the patient likely contagious?
   a. 1 week
   b. 2 weeks
   c. 4 weeks
   d. 8 weeks

159. A 66-year-old male patient has increasing abdominal pain and has been passing 3 to 4 sticky, black, foul-smelling stools for 3 to 4 days. The patient's vital signs are BP 116/78 mm Hg supine, pulse rate 112 bpm, respiratory rate of 22 breaths/minute, and temperature 37°C (98.6°F). Standing BP dropped to 88/58 mm Hg, and the patient experienced dizziness. The patient's hemoglobin is 9.2 mg/dL (92 mmol/L), hematocrit 28%, MCV 90 fL, and BUN 46 mg/dL (16.4 mmol/L). Based on these observations, the CNS should suspect
   a. iron deficiency anemia and intestinal perforation.
   b. hemolytic anemia and gastritis.
   c. iron deficiency anemia and upper GI bleeding.
   d. iron deficiency anemia and lower GI bleeding.

160. A patient with multiple sclerosis tells the nurse that she is upset that she can no longer continue her employment because her job is too physically demanding and she is concerned about how she will support herself. Which of the following responses focuses on problem solving as a response to stress?
   a. "What plans do you have for finding a new job?"
   b. "You might be eligible for public assistance."
   c. "I'm sure there is other work you can do."
   d. "I can see how upsetting that is for you."

161. A patient who recently returned from serving in the military in the Middle East is hospitalized with post-traumatic stress disorder. The patient has recurring flashbacks and nightmares and is constantly vigilant and anxious. The patient tells the CNS repeatedly that he should have died with his friends. Which of the following is the *most appropriate* response?
   a. "You have a lot to live for."
   b. "You won't always feel that way, I'm sure."
   c. "Why do you feel that way?"
   d. "Are you thinking about killing yourself?"

162. The CNS is screening patients for referral to a case manager. Which of the following patients is *most* likely to benefit from case management?
   a. an 18-year-old patient with second-degree burns on the hands
   b. a 62-year-old patient with repeated hospitalizations for COPD and diabetes
   c. a 38-year-old patient post-mastectomy for breast cancer
   d. a 52-year old patient post knee replacement

163. The CNS is supervising a novice nurse. Which of the following actions by the nurse should cause the CNS to intervene?
   a. The nurse works more slowly than more experienced nurses.
   b. The nurse frequently asks for advice about care planning.
   c. The nurse administers medications without checking patient IDs.
   d. The nurse checks the procedure manual before carrying out procedures.

164. When the CNS is researching evidence-based practice, which research design provides the *best* information about cause and effect relationships?
   a. one group, post-test only
   b. crossover/Counterbalancing
   c. descriptive
   d. randomized controlled trials

165. The CNS is teaching a patient with amyotrophic lateral sclerosis (ALS) to manage the disease. Which of the following is an example of the CNS using the tool of *negotiating*?
   a. CNS presents the pros and cons of treatment.
   b. CNS utilizes motivational interviewing.
   c. CNS helps patient to obtain information.
   d. CNS conducts follow-up with patient.

166. The CNS is preparing patient education materials as part of a series of health classes being offered to patients with chronic illness. When developing instructional materials, the 3 major components that the CNS must consider are the
   a. cost, time, and effort.
   b. delivery system, content, and presentation.
   c. simplicity, effectiveness, and content.
   d. cost, delivery system, and content.

167. The CNS has proposed use of the SBAR format for hand-off communication but is encountering resistance from long-time staff members who dislike change. The *best* method of dealing with resistance is to
   a. ignore the complaints.
   b. inform resistant staff members that they are impeding process.
   c. encourage staff to express opinions and discuss concerns.
   d. propose a vote regarding the use of SBAR.

168. The CNS is giving an interview to a reporter of a local newspaper about a community health prevention program that the CNS is spearheading. The CNS should
   a. avoid scientific jargon.
   b. suggest a story angle.
   c. ask for a prepublication copy of article.
   d. discuss only positive aspects of the program.

169. A patient with dilated cardiomyopathy is on the transplant list for a heart but none has become available. The patient's ejection fraction has fallen to 22%, and the patient's functional ability is markedly decreased. The CNS recognizes that the patient may benefit most from a(n)
   a. pacemaker.
   b. LVAD.
   c. IABP.
   d. ICD.

170. When analyzing data as part of clinical research, the CNS includes only those cases that relate specifically to the requirement of the measurement and excludes cases that are similar but associated with a different population in order to decrease the number of false positive. The issue that the CNS is addressing is
 a. sensitivity.
 b. reliability.
 c. specificity.
 d. validity.

171. According to NANDA guidelines, which of the following is an example of a problem-focused nursing diagnosis?
 a. Risk of aspiration as evidenced by dysphagia and impaired cough reflex.
 b. Risk of DVT as evidenced by immobility and peripheral edema.
 c. Readiness for discharge as evidenced by independence in self-care.
 d. Pain related to abdominal incision with inflammation (erythema, edema) as evidenced by verbalization of pain, guarding, and social withdrawal.

172. A patient with chronic low back pain states he wants to try complementary theapy to relieve pain as medications have been ineffective and asks CNS which of the therapies are likely to relieve discomfort. The CNS should reply that therapy that has documented effectiveness is
 a. acupuncture.
 b. herbal medicines.
 c. homeopathic medicines.
 d. healing touch.

173. Which of the following is the most important factor in determining whether an event is a stressor to a patient?
 a. patient's education
 b. patient age
 c. patient's perception
 d. patient's support system

174. If a CNS was exposed to tuberculosis at work and developed active pulmonary TB, the CNS must be excluded from work until treatment is completed OR
 a. 1 sputum test is negative.
 b. 2 sputum tests are negative.
 c. 3 sputum tests are negative.
 d. 4 sputum tests are negative.

175. If the CNS hears a patient's physician complaining that a patient is "difficult and impatient," and the CNS tells the physician that the patient is very frightened and acting defensively, the aspect of care that the nurse is exhibiting is
 a. advocacy.
 b. patient equality.
 c. human dignity preservation.
 d. caring practice.

# Answers and Explanations

1. **D**: If the CNS is caring for a patient who has a history of cocaine abuse, the health problems for which the CNS should be alert include nasal sores and septal perforation (from snorting the drug) and cardiac dysrhythmias. The patient may also develop chronic sinusitis. Opioid use is characterized by sexual dysfunction, gastric ulcers, and glomerulonephritis. Amphetamines may result in uncontrolled tremors, cardiac dysrhythmias, and impaired cognition; sedative/hypnotics may result in memory impairment and respiratory depression.

2. **B**: If, according to his son, a 70-year-old man whose wife died 6 months earlier appeared to grieve little and manage well after her death, resuming an active social life, but has become increasingly withdrawn in the past month, eating and sleeping poorly and wandering the house at night, resulting in hospitalization for depression, the priority intervention for the CNS should be to encourage the patient to talk about his wife and her death. The patient is likely having a delayed grief response and dysfunctional grieving.

3. **C**: If a patient is on bedrest with myocarditis, the toileting option that the CNS should recommend is usually the use of a bedside commode. While rest is critical for healing of the cardiac muscle, using a bedpan is likely to induce more stress on the heart than getting out of bed to use the commode. The patient should be assisted to sitting position and onto the commode, which should be placed adjacent to the bed.

4. **A**: If a 33-year-old woman is hospitalized for treatment of acute pyelonephritis and has been receiving IV fluids and ampicillin plus aminoglycoside for the past 5 days but her temperature remains elevated and she is still in pain and nauseated, she should likely be evaluated for perinephric abscess. With perinephric abscess, the onset of symptoms is usually slower than with acute pyelonephritis, and fever often persists for more than 4 days.

5. **D**: If a patient who suffered a stroke has persistent dysphagia and cough and the CNS is concerned that the patient may aspirate, the most appropriate referral is to a speech pathologist. The speech pathologist is able to assess the strength of the mouth, including the lips, the tongue, the palate, and the jaw. The speech pathologist may suggest preventive measures, including positioning and diet modifications, and may prescribe exercises and/or neurological stimulation or thermostimulation.

6. **C**: If a 56-year-old patient is admitted for possible pancreatitis, the laboratory tests that are needed on admission to apply Ranson's criteria are WBC, glucose, AST, and LDH. One point is awarded for each item; at least 3 points is predicted mortality of 11% to 15% and at least 6 points is 40%:

| Ranson's Criteria for Predicting Severity of Pancreatitis | |
|---|---|
| **Criteria on admission** | **Criteria within 48 hours** |
| <ul><li>Age > 55 years</li><li>WBC > 16,000/mcL</li><li>Glucose > 200 mg/dL (10 mmol/L)</li><li>AST > 250 U/L (4.25 microkat/L)</li><li>LDH > 350 U/L</li></ul> | <ul><li>Hematocrit drop > 10% from admission</li><li>BUN increase > 5 mg/dL (> 1.7 mmol/L) despite fluids</li><li>Calcium < 8 mg/dL (< 2 mmol/L)</li><li>Arterial pO$_2$ < 60 mm Hg</li><li>Base deficit > 4 mEq/L</li><li>Fluid requirement > 6 L</li></ul> |

7. B: If the CNS works with a population that includes males having sex with males (MSM), the CNS should recommend the HPV vaccination for MSM equal to or younger than 26 years because infections associated with HPV, including anogenital warts and anal squamous intraepithelial lesions, are common in this population. MSM should also be screened for other STDs, including HIV, syphilis, gonorrhea, and chlamydia, at least annually. Patients should be advised to use condoms for every sexual encounter.

8. A: If a 28-year-old patient with 3 young children has ovarian cancer and is to be discharged to her home with fentanyl transdermal patches for pain control, when teaching the patient about the use of the patches, the CNS should stress that discarded patches must be folded and immediately flushed down the toilet. Used patches still contain the opioid and can result in overdose and death of small children who come in contact with them; they are also a grave risk to drug seekers who smoke discarded patches.

9. D: If a 76-year-old woman ate *E.coli* (O157:H7)–contaminated vegetables and developed abdominal cramps and non-bloody diarrhea that persisted for 48 hours, after which the diarrhea became bloody and has remained so for 4 days, if the condition does not resolve, she is at risk of developing hemolytic uremic syndrome (HUS), which can lead to renal failure. Children younger than 5 years and older adults are most likely to develop HUS. HUS is characterized by microangiopathic hemolytic anemia, thrombocytopenia, and acute renal failure.

10. A: If the CNS is conducting clinical research and intends to select participants that will be able to provide a particular perspective related to the research question, this type of sampling is referred to as purposeful because selection is based on the needs of the study. Nominated sampling enrolls participants through recommendations of those already enrolled. Convenience or volunteer sampling requires finding participants through solicitation or advertising. Theoretical sampling is a form of purposeful sample that uses participants to build a theory.

11. B: If the CNS is leading an ad hoc team that is utilizing failure mode and effects analysis (FMEA) to identify potential failures in the system that may result in increased healthcare-associated infections, once a list of potential failures is complied, calculation of the risk priority number (RPN) (S X O X D = RPN) is based on:
- Severity: Each potential failure is rated on a scale of 1 to 10 (1 equal to a slight problem and 10 equal to death).
- Occurrence: Each potential failure is rated on a scale of 1 to 10 according to the likelihood that the failure will occur within a specified period of time (such as a year).
- Detection: Each potential failure is rated on a scale of 1 to 10 according to the likelihood that the problem will be detected before it occurs.

12. A: The statement by a patient that indicates that the CNS needs to provide education is: "I take all kinds of herbal medicines because I know they're always safe." The CNS should advise the patient that herbal medicines can interact with prescribed medicines, so the patient should always discuss herbal medicines with healthcare providers before taking them and be sure to follow directions regarding recommended dosages. Additionally, some herbal preparations can cause serious adverse effects.

13. D: If a 49-year-old man has severe chest pain radiating to left shoulder and arm, and vital signs include BP 152/92 mm Hg, pulse rate of 96 bpm, respiratory rate 20 breaths/minute, oxygen saturation 94%, and temperature 38°C (100.4°F), and he is nauseated, his skin is clammy, and his ECG shows anterior STEMI, the treatment priority should include aspirin (ASA) 324 mg and a

nitrate sublingually every 5 minutes as needed up to 15 minutes. If the nitrate is ineffective in relieving pain, then morphine should be administered. Oxygen may be necessary, although oxygen saturation at 94% is only slightly outside normal parameters (95% to 100%).

14. C: If a 64-year-old female patient has persistent overflow incontinence resulting from an areflexic detrusor muscle, the treatment that the CNS should recommend is intermittent catheterization if the patient is able to carry out the procedure. A Foley catheter may be inserted but increases the risk of infection because colonization of bacteria usually occurs within 14 days. A Foley catheter should be routinely changed at least once monthly as encrustations may cause blockage and bladder spasms.

15. B: If the CNS is working on a unit that has been understaffed and one of the nurses on the unit states that his blood pressure has increased because he dreads coming to work and feels that the organization does not value nurses or care about patients and that nothing will change, the CNS should recognize that the nurse is most at risk for burnout. Stages of stress include:
    1. fight or flight response
    2. emotional reaction: anger, shock, surprise
    3. negative thinking
    4. physical reaction
    5. no change in stressor or person
    6. burnout.

16. D: When the CNS is delegating a task, the delegation process should begin with the task to be delegated and the expected outcomes. The CNS should identify priorities if a number of steps or tasks are involved and advise the other team members of monitoring that the CNS may carry out as well as any specific time frame that may be necessary for completion of the task. The team members should be aware of reporting parameters, such as critical information that must be reported immediately.

17. A: If the CNS walks by a patient's room and notes that the patient's upper side rails are elevated and the patient's bed in high position while the patient is unattended, the CNS should lower the bed, immediately resolving the safety issue, and discuss safety issues with staff members, including the importance of keeping beds in the low position unless actively caring for the patient. This type of safety issue is rarely intentional, so trying to assign blame serves little useful purpose.

18. B: A realistic goal to be included in the care plan of a patient with diabetes mellitus is A1c of less than 7%. Other goals should include maintaining a preprandial glucose level of 70 to 130 mg/dL (3.9 to 7.2 mmol/L) and a peak postprandial glucose level of less than 180 mg/dL (10 mmol/L). While these goals are ideal, they may need to be modified for the individual patient, depending on the severity of diabetes, comorbidities, age, and other factors.

19. C: A patient newly diagnosed with tuberculosis and taking isoniazid (INH) should take vitamin $B_6$ (pyridoxine) with the INH to prevent peripheral neuropathy. The patient should be advised to take medications exactly as prescribed and to avoid alcoholic beverages during treatment. The patient should also have a good understanding of adverse effects associated with anti-tubercular treatment and advise healthcare providers of any other medications the patient is prescribed or taking because of possible drug interactions.

20. D: If the CNS is promoting evidence-based practice and using the PICOT format to pose a clinical question, the CNS would first focus on the patient population. PICOT:

| PICOT format | |
|---|---|
| Patient population | What is the target population (adults, children, homeless) or setting (home care, inpatient, outpatient)? |
| Intervention/Area of interest | What is the potential intervention? |
| Comparison | What are other interventions? |
| Outcome | What are strategies for measuring outcomes? |
| Time | What is the time frame for intervention? |

21. A: If a patient being treated for endocarditis has developed sudden onset of hematuria, the CNS should alert the physician regarding possible renal embolization. Embolization is a high risk during the first 3 months of treatment and may result in stroke, pulmonary embolus, and splenic embolization as well as renal embolization. Endocarditis can result from bacteremia, transient or chronic, and may occur in patients who are IV drug users or those with prosthetic heart disease, rheumatic heart disease, mitral valve prolapse, and other cardiac abnormalities.

22. B: If a volunteer who is a native speaker of the language of a priority population translated materials for a health education program for the CNS without being asked, the CNS should verify the translations with a professional translator before using the materials. People's ability to translate varies widely and even one wrong word or phrase may substantially alter the meaning. If a local translator is not available, translation services are often available through the Internet.

23. C: If the CNS is conducting classes regarding infection control, the following are included:
- Goals: Increase compliance with handwashing standards.
- Objectives: Observe 100% compliance with handwashing.
- Strategies: Place handwashing posters in all nursing units.
- Lesson plans: Discussion period—The nurse's role in reducing infection.

The goal is the overall purpose of the class while the objectives should be measurable as they are used to determine if the purpose has been met. Strategies are the methods used and lesson plans are the specific way the material is presented.

24. D: If a patient is undergoing thrombolytic infusion for pulmonary emboli and must have a venipuncture for laboratory tests, manual pressure should be applied to the venipuncture site for at least 30 minutes because the anticoagulation may result in prolonged bleeding. The patient must be carefully monitored during thrombolytic therapy with vital signs assessed frequently. The patient should remain on bedrest. The patient's INR and PTT are generally checked 3 to 4 hours after the infusion is completed.

25. B: If a 70-year-old woman with COPD has experienced an exacerbation after contracting an upper respiratory infection and her oxygen saturation level is 84%, pH 7.29, $PaCO_2$ 52 mm Hg, $PaO_2$ 53 mm Hg, and $HCO_3$ 25 mEq/L, the acid-base imbalance that the patient is experiencing is respiratory acidosis. The pH is acidotic (< 7.35), the $PaCO_2$ is elevated (normal 35 to 45 mm Hg), and the $PaO_2$ is at the low end of normal (normal ≥ 80 mm Hg), indicating the problem is respiratory in nature. The $HCO_3$ remains within normal range but near the upper limit (normal 22 to 26 mEq/L). These findings indicate a sudden decrease in ventilation.

26. A: If the CNS works with a group of ethnically diverse staff members, but a number of conflicts have arisen because of different methods of communication and attitudes toward authority, the best solution is likely to initiate a discussion about cultural differences, including direct versus indirect communication. Ignoring the situation or issuing guidelines is not likely to alter the situation unless the problem is dealt with directly by those involved. Through discussion, better approaches to communication may develop.

27. D: If a 27-year-old male patient has had increased thirst and frequency of urination, including nocturia, increased appetite but recent weight loss and laboratory tests show glucose of 526 mg/dL (29.2 mmol/L), urine positive for glucose and ketones, and blood pH of 7.22 (normal 7.35 to 7.45), the blood pH is the result of increased ketone levels in the blood. Because insulin supply is inadequate and glucose level high, the body breaks down fat to use as a source of energy. As the blood lipid level increases, these lipids are metabolized, resulting in ketones as byproducts, including acetoacetic acid and beta-hydroxybutyric acid. These acidic byproducts increase acidity of the blood.

28. C: If the CNS needs to interview a patient who is lying supine in bed because of a back injury, the best means of ensuring a therapeutic interaction is for the CNS to pull up a chair and sit at bedside. This puts the CNS at approximately the same level as the patient, facilitating eye contact and interactions. The CNS should avoid power positions, such as standing and looking down on the patient, if possible.

29. A: If a 24-year-old patient diagnosed with type 1 diabetes mellitus with a glucose level of 468 mg/dL (26 mmol/L), polyuria, polydipsia, and weight loss has stabilized since starting insulin injections and now appears to be able to manage the diabetes with very little insulin, the CNS should suspect that the patient's insulin needs will increase again. Symptoms of diabetes usually do not occur until about destruction of 90% of the pancreatic islet. Once stabilized, the patient often undergoes a "honeymoon" period when the remaining cells seem to produce enough insulin, but the same process of cell destruction and increased blood glucose will continue.

30. D: If the CNS is collaborating with the public health department in an initiative to collect data about community needs, the first step should be to define the population. For example, the target population may be one particular ethnic group (such as Mexican immigrants), one social group (the homeless), or a population in one area (rural, urban, suburban). A decision should be made whether the entire population should be targeted or a sampling of the larger population.

31. C: If a 32-year old woman reports 6 to 10 episodes of palpitation daily, irritability, insomnia, heat intolerance, eye irritation, increased appetite coupled with weight loss; vital signs are BP 170/86 mm Hg, pulse 114 bpm, respiratory rate of 20 breaths/minute, and temperature 37.5°C (99.5°F), and ECG shows atrial fibrillation, the patient should undergo thyroid function tests (T3, T4, and TSH) as these signs and symptoms are indicative of hyperthyroidism. Hyperthyroidism may be associated with Graves disease (an autoimmune disorder), thyroiditis, or pituitary tumors.

32. B: If a 19-year-old female patient with sickle cell disease experienced an aplastic crisis and has a hemoglobin of 5.6 g/dL (56 mmol/L), she will likely receive transfusions of packed red blood cells until her hemoglobin reaches 10 g/dL (100 mmol/L). Hemoglobin levels of 6 to 9 g/dL (60 to 90 mmol/L) are common in patients with sickle cell disease because their RBC survive only 10 to 12 days rather than the 120 that is normal.

33. A: If a 46-year-old patient suffered blood loss in a motor vehicle accident and the patient's hemoglobin is 14.1 g/dL (141 mmol/L) and hematocrit 43%, ECG shows slight ST depression, BUN is 32 mg/dL (11.42 mmol/L), creatinine 2.5 mg/dL (221 micromol/L), ALT 42 U/L and AST 49 U/L (0.83 microkat/L), these findings most likely represent hypovolemia and liver ischemia. Hemoglobin and hematocrit remain stable initially, but the elevated BUN and creatinine indicate that blood flow to the kidneys is impaired, suggestive of hypovolemia. The elevated ALT and ST indicate that circulation of blood to the liver is impaired, resulting in ischemia.

34. D: If a 78-year-old patient with COPD is hospitalized with acute respiratory distress syndrome (ARDS), pronounced wheezing, fever (38.6°C [101.5°F]), and cough; and arterial blood gases are pH 7.24, $PaO_2$ 49 mm Hg, and $PaCO_2$ 61 mm Hg, and the patient is provided steroids and bronchodilators, is alert and able to follow directions but unable to speak because of dyspnea, the treatment that is most appropriate to relieve respiratory distress is non-invasive ventilation (NIV). NIV does not require intubation but delivers forced air through a facemask, nasal mask, or helmet mask.

35. C: While asthma attacks and COPD exacerbations may be difficult to distinguish based on x-rays, signs and symptoms, and laboratory tests, some characteristics can help to distinguish the two:
   - Onset of asthma is at a younger age, usually younger than 30 years, than COPD, which most often occurs after age 40.
   - Asthma attacks can usually be fairly quickly resolved with treatment, but COPD responds more slowly and often only temporarily.
   - Asthma has a genetic component, but COPD generally does not.
   - Asthma patients are much less likely to have been smokers while almost all COPD patients have smoked.

36. B: Sudden lumbar pain radiating to the flank and groin area may be an indication that an abdominal aortic aneurysm rupture is imminent as the pain occurs as the aneurysm begins to rapidly enlarge. This is an emergent situation that requires immediate surgical repair. If the aneurysm ruptures and hemorrhaging into the peritoneal cavity occurs, the patient may have severe abdominal and/or back pain. If the aneurysm ruptures into the duodenum, massive GI bleeding may occur.

37. C: If a patient was hit in the head with a hard ball and lost consciousness for a brief period but was then alert and responsive but became unstable 2 hours later with severe headache, visual disturbances, nausea and vomiting, and seizures, the patient should undergo a CT to confirm a possible epidural hematoma. An MRI may also provide accurate information, but it requires longer and is not recommended for unstable patients. Angiography may be indicated for some patients. X-rays provide information only about overlying skull fractures.

38. D: If a patient who was a victim of a violent assault and rape is shaking and crying and appears terrified, the most therapeutic response at the time of the initial encounter with the patient is, "You are safe now." The patient is likely still in the "fight or flight" mode with increased adrenaline from having to deal with the assault and rape, police intervention, and now a medical examination, so it is important for the CNS to provide calm reassurance to the patient to try to allay fears.

39. B: The teaching strategy that is the most efficient approach for a group of 8 patients regarding the need for lifestyle changes needed to manage hypertension and heart disease is lecture-discussion. This format allows the CNS to provide information in a short lecture format and then provides the patients with time to ask questions and discuss the information shared. Supplemental

printed materials may be provided to the patients. The CNS should cover no more than 5 to 7 different topics in one session.

40. A: If the CNS examines a patient's functional ability and notes that the patient's gait is characterized by shuffling of the feet with periodic short rapid steps while the neck, trunk, and knees are flexed and the patient leans forward, increasingly walking faster, the CNS should recognize this gait as characteristic of Parkinson disease. The patient may also exhibit a blank facial expression, slow monotonous or slurred speech, and tremors. Classic manifestations include the triad of tremor, rigidity, and bradykinesia.

41. C: If, when conducting a history and physical exam of a patient with dyspnea, the CNS discovers that the patient has smoked 1.5 packs (30) cigarettes daily for at least 15 years, this represents 30 pack-years. One pack-year is equal to smoking 1 pack (20) of cigarettes daily for a year. The greater the number of pack-years, the higher the risk of developing COPD. Most patients with COPD have smoked for 40 pack-years, and symptoms are not usually evident until more than 20 pack-years of smoking.

42. D: If a patient has fractured ribs that resulted in a left pneumothorax of about 12%, the CNS should anticipate that the treatment will include supplementary oxygen only and observation unless the pneumothorax increases over 15%. With a larger pneumothorax, a needle aspiration may be done and either a small bore (12 to 20 Fr) or a large bore (24 to 40 Fr) chest tube inserted. The chest tube is then attached to a Heimlich one-way valve that allows air to leave the pleural space but not to enter or to an underwater seal system.

43. C: If a patient with HIV/AIDS and a history of drug abuse has moved home with aging parents who are not supportive, and he requires assistance with ADLS and treatment, frequently misses appointments, and fails to follow treatment regimen, the patient's characteristic is best described as complex. Multiple factors are at play (family dynamics, patient's HIV status, patient's depression, treatment requirements) and must be considered when assisting the patient with the plan of care.

44. B: If a patient with a suspected brain tumor exhibits lack of coordination, memory loss, and speech difficulties, the most likely tumor location is the temporal lobe. A tumor in the frontal lobe may result in mood and personality changes as well as hemiparesis. A tumor in the parietal lobe may cause impaired sensation and loss of fine motor skills and half-body awareness. A tumor in the occipital lobe may cause vision disturbances and visual hallucinations. Cerebellar tumors affect coordination and balance while brain stem tumors result in cranial nerve dysfunction, facial pain, and dysphagia.

45. A: If a patient experiencing an acute episode of asthma is anxious, sitting in tripod position with audible wheezing resulting from upper airway obstruction with a peak flow of 65% of normal and oxygen saturation of 92%, the initial treatment should be the rescue protocol that generally begins with an inhaled short-acting beta-2 agonist, such as albuterol (Proventil HFA), to relax smooth muscles. An anticholinergic, such as ipratropium bromide (Atrovent HFA), may also be given to relieve bronchospasm. If there is no improvement within 10 minutes, then prednisone or methylprednisolone is usually administered.

46. D: If a patient with acute pericarditis has severe sternal pain radiating to the neck and increasing on inspiration, the CNS should advise the patient to sit up and lean forward. This position allows the heart to pull slightly away from the diaphragmatic pleurae, relieving some of the discomfort. The patient should be carefully assessed because increased pain, especially if

accompanied by pallor, hypotension, paradoxical pulse, dyspnea, and/or jugular venous distention, may indicate cardiac tamponade.

47. B: If a 60-year-old African American patient has a BMI of 32 kg/m², hemoglobin A1C level of 7.1 (71 mmol/L), fasting serum glucose 152 mg/dL (8.4mmol/L), triglyceride level of 168 and HDL 24 mg/dL, and the patient is diagnosed with insulin resistance and diabetes mellitus, type 2, the drug of choice for initiating therapy is usually a biguanide, typically metformin. Metformin is usually tolerated well and does not cause hypoglycemia. If the A1c levels have not fallen to below 7% within about 3 months, an additional medication is prescribed.

48. D: According to the WHO three-step ladder approach to pain management, if a patient's abdominal pain associated with pancreatic cancer varies from 4 to 8 on the pain scale, pain control should be initiated at whichever step is most appropriate for the level of pain at the time and then may later be adjusted to a higher or lower step. While this is a three-step process, it is not necessary to start all pain control at step one.

49. C: If a patient under hospice care for end-of-life care for stage 4 multiple myeloma has developed severe skeletal pain and is scheduled to undergo radiation therapy to reduce discomfort, this treatment does not affect hospice care because although radiation may be an active treatment in some cases, the intent of the treatment is to provide palliation rather than to delay disease progress or to cure the disease. While there is no preauthorization process for treatment under hospice, there are appeal processes that are utilized after hospice service has been denied.

50. A: Following lunch, if a 72-year-old woman experiences a sudden episode of loss of vision in the right eye during which she feels dizzy and weak, and her speech is slightly garbled, but the symptoms clear within 15 to 20 minutes, the most likely diagnosis is transient ischemic episode (TIE). Transient impaired vision of one eye (amaurosis fugax) is a common finding with TIE, which is often a precursor to a stroke; the patient should undergo a complete examination.

51. C: If a patient being treated for cardiogenic shock after an acute myocardial infarction has an IABP in place and the radiology technician has arrived in the unit to take a portable chest x-ray to evaluate the degree of pulmonary edema, when the CNS observes the technician preparing to sit the patient upright in order to place the cassette film hold behind the patient's back, the CNS should immediately stop the technician. If the patient is placed in sitting position when the balloon is inflated, the pressure can cause rupture of the aorta. Additionally, the patient should not flex the hips as this may damage or displace the catheter.

52. C: If a patient is admitted to the ED for an ischemic stroke, the most essential laboratory tests prior to thrombolysis are the glucose level and coagulation studies. Patients with hypoglycemia may have clinical indications that are similar to those experienced with a stroke, so the level should be above 50 mg/dL (2.8 mmol/L). Hyperglycemia can worsen the effects of the stroke and result in a poor outcome, so treatment may include insulin to bring glucose level to less than 140 mg/dL (7.8 mmol/L). Coagulation studies must be done to assess risk of bleeding with thrombolysis.

53. B: If a patient involved in a motor vehicle accident has bruising over the area of the mastoid process (Battle's sign) as well as bilateral "raccoon eyes" (swollen ecchymotic), the injuries are consistent with the clinical signs of a basilar skull fracture. Basilar skull fractures may occur with impact to the occipital or mandibular areas or may extend from fractures of the cranial vault. Patients may also develop rhinorrhea or otorrhea from leakage of cerebrospinal fluid through the torn dural membrane.

54. D: The patient most at risk of development of a chronic subdural hematoma 3 to 4 weeks after initial injury is the 78-year-old patient who fell and hit the head on the floor but experienced only a slight headache at the time. Chronic subdural hematomas are most common in elderly patients, probably because atrophy of the brain allows for more movement during injury, and this can tear vessels. In many cases, patients do not recall any prior injury.

55. A: The AVPU assessment is done after a head injury to determine the patient's level of consciousness. This is a rapid assessment tool used when initially examining a patient.

| AVPU | | | |
|---|---|---|---|
| A | Alert and awake, oriented to person, place, time, and condition | Yes | No |
| V | Responds to verbal stimuli | Yes | No |
| P | Responds to painful stimuli but not verbal | Yes | No |
| U | Unconscious, does not respond to painful or verbal stimuli | Yes | No |

56. A: If the medical-surgical unit has experienced an outbreak of *Clostridium difficile* infections involving 10 patients over a 2-week period, in order the reduce transmission of the infection, the CNS is working with staff members and should concentrate efforts on the utilization of proper contact precautions and hand hygiene as the infection is easily spread through contaminated hands. The spores can remain viable on environmental surfaces for long periods of time. Housekeeping procedures should also be reviewed.

57. B: If a patient was stung by a bee and has pain and itching around the site of the bee sting with erythema and edema extending about 8 cm diameter around the site, but the patient has no systemic manifestations, the initial medication should be an antihistamine, such as diphenhydramine (Benadryl). Diphenhydramine will help to control local allergic response and to relieve itching. A topical corticosteroid may also be applied to relieve itching. Epinephrine and corticosteroids are reserved for systemic reactions and those at risk of anaphylaxis.

58. C: Using the Rule of 9s, if a patient has burns from toxic chemicals covering the chest (but not the abdomen) and the anterior surface of the left arm, the BSA with burns is approximately 13.5%. Each arm accounts for about 9%, with 4.5% for the anterior surface and 4.5% for the posterior surface. The anterior trunk covers 18%, but since only the chest was burned, this is 9%. The BSA of the back is 18% and each leg is 18%, with 9% for the anterior surface and 9% for the posterior. The genital area is 1%.

59. D: If a patient involved in a motor vehicle accident had multiple injuries, including fractured ribs, an unstable posterior ring pelvic fracture, and blunt liver trauma, and received transfusions, external fixation of pelvic fracture, and nonoperative management of liver trauma, during the recovery period, the patient is most at risk of deep vein thrombosis and pulmonary embolus. Once the patient has stabilized, DVT prophylaxis, such as warfarin or low-molecular-weight heparin, may be administered. The patient should be mobilized as quickly as possible.

60. A: If a patient developed SIADH after taking sertraline, which is associated with hyponatremia, and her serum sodium level is 120 mEq/L (120 mmol/L), and she exhibits mild confusion, anorexia, and nausea, in addition to discontinuation of the sertraline, the first-line intervention is to limit fluid intake. Severe neurological damage can occur if the sodium level is increased too rapidly, so

the patient must be carefully monitored. Normal values for serum sodium are 135 to 145 mEq/L (135 to 145 mmol/L) with hyponatremia of less than 120 mEq/L (120 mmol/L) a critical finding.

61. B: If an older patient tells the CNS that she is very concerned that her end-of-life care provides comfort and avoids unnecessary interventions, the best recommendation for the patient is to prepare an advance directive that outlines in detail the type of end-of-life care the patient wants. The patient should also be advised to share the advance directive with family members because in most states, if the patient is incapacitated, the advance directive is not legally binding and may be overridden by family members.

62. D: If a patient is admitted to the hospital with a diagnosis of left ventricular heart failure, the CNS should expect the clinical indications to include dyspnea and cough as well a generalized weakness and fatigue. With left-sided failure, the left ventricle becomes enlarged because of increased workload and end-diastolic volume. The impaired function results in blood pooling in the ventricles and backing up into the pulmonary veins, resulting in engorgement of the pulmonary circulation and pulmonary edema.

63. C: If a patient's cardiac monitor shows the following heart pattern, the CNS should recognize this ECG recording as ventricular fibrillation (VF) and anticipate that the patient will require defibrillation. With VF, the ventricular rate may be greater than 300 beats per minute with no atrial activity observable. If no pulse is palpable or audible, then VF is life-threatening. VF may occur if ventricular tachycardia is left untreated. VF may also result from electrical shock as well as coronary artery disease. It may be triggered by caffeine or nicotine.

64. B: If a patient with end-stage renal disease develops a hypertensive crisis with BP of 182/108 mm Hg, heart rate 104 bpm, respirations 18 breaths/minute, and oxygen saturation of 98%, and the patient is anxious and complains of headache but there is no indication of organ damage, this type of hypertensive crisis is categorized as a hypertensive urgency. The patient must be monitored closely while receiving labetalol because the blood pressure must be reduced slowly to avoid hypotension and ischemia of internal organs. Reduction should be about 33% in the first 6 hours, 33% in the next 24 hours, and 33% over the next 2 to 4 days.

65. D: If a patient is recovering from CABG and ambulating in the hallway with a wireless cardiac monitor when an alarm sounds indicating that the patient is experiencing supraventricular tachycardia with a pulse rate of 162 bpm, the priority intervention should be to assist the patient to sit down as she is at risk of falling, and activity may further stress the heart. Then, the nurse should take the patient's blood pressure if it is not evident on the monitor and notify the physician. As soon as possible, the patient should be placed in a wheelchair (if not already in one) and moved to the bed in the patient's room.

66. A: If a post-anesthesia patient just awakening following removal of the intubation tube begins to cough and aspiration of gastric fluids is suspected, the CNS should immediately lower the patient's head and turn the patient to the side so that secretions in the trachea can drain out by gravity. The focus of treatment is on ensuring tissue oxygenation. The patient may receive supplemental oxygen and CPAP or non-invasive ventilation (NIV). In some cases, the patient may need to be reintubated for mechanical ventilation.

67. B: If a patient with heart failure has developed pulmonary edema and has rales and rhonchi present throughout the lungs fields and is very anxious, and initial treatment includes 15 L oxygen per non-rebreather mask, furosemide 60 mg IV, nitroglycerine, nitroprusside, and morphine to reduce anxiety, the initial goal of therapy should be to maintain the PaO$_2$ above 60 mm Hg. While the normal PaO$_2$ ranges from 80 to 95 mm Hg, the critical value is below 45 mm Hg, at which point perfusion is inadequate.

68. A: If a 64-year-old African American male patient with diabetes has BP readings that average about 154/96 mm Hg, the first-line pharmacologic therapy that the CNS should advise is a thiazide diuretic or calcium channel blocker. If a patient is of a different ethnic group, the initial therapy may include a thiazide diuretic, calcium channel blocker, ACE inhibitor, or ARB. If the patient does not respond adequately to the first drug, most often a thiazide diuretic, then a second drug and, in some cases, a third drug should be added. ACE inhibitors should not be given with ARBs.

69. B: If a 56-year-old patient experienced blunt thoracic trauma during a motor vehicle accident at 20 mph, the most appropriate initial diagnostic tool to assess for cardiac trauma is an ECG. Patients who are older than 50 years and traveling at speeds over 15 mph are especially at risk. Blunt cardiac trauma may result in various dysrhythmias, but the most common finding is sinus tachycardia. If the ECG is abnormal and the patient is hemodynamically unstable, than an echocardiogram should be obtained.

70. C: If following cardiac surgery for repair of aortic valve, the patient has acute chest pain and shortness of breath, relieved by sitting up and learning forward, and the patient is diaphoretic and hypotensive with weak and rapid peripheral pulses and paradoxical pulse and narrow pulse pressure, the CNS should prepare the patient for emergent pericardiocentesis. These signs and symptoms are characteristic of cardiac tamponade, and failure to recognize the signs and respond immediately may result in pulseless electrical activity (PEA) and death.

71. A: The interaction between the CNS and a patient of a different ethnic and cultural background that indicates the CNS's cultural responsiveness is when the CNS discusses the purpose and meaning of the medical regimen. A patient should not feel that treatment is imposed but should be actively involved in the plan of care and should be encouraged to ask questions and relate the treatment to ethnic and cultural practices so that the patient is more likely to adhere to the regimen.

72. A: If a patient is taking atorvastatin for dyslipidemia, a bile acid sequestrant may be recommended for its additive effect to reduce the risk of cardiac mortality resulting from dyslipidemia. Bile acid sequestrants are resins that bind bile acids and prevent reabsorption and are effective in lowering LDL cholesterol. They are sometimes used along with statins. Fibrates should be avoided because combining them with statins may result in increased risk of rhabdomyolysis.

73. D: If a patient with acute respiratory failure (ARF) is intubated and receiving mechanical ventilation, one of the steps to preventing ventilator-associated pneumonia (VAP) is to provide DVT prophylaxis as the immobility increases risk of DVT and pulmonary emboli. Other steps include keeping the head of the bed elevated to at least 30 degrees, reducing sedation for a period daily to determine if the patient is ready for extubation, providing daily oral care with chlorhexidine, and peptic ulcer prophylaxis to reduce the risk of aspiration.

74. B: If a patient has increasing intracranial pressure (ICP), the aim of treatment is to maintain the ICP at less than 20 mm Hg. Normal values vary but usually range from 5 to 15 mm Hg. Treatment is usually conservative if pressure is between 15 to 20 mm Hg, but pressure of greater than 20 mm Hg (usually with Glasgow Coma Scale [GCS] of 8 or less) may result in damage to the brain tissue, compression of structures, and herniation syndrome.

75. B: If a patient with multiple anterior and posterior coronary artery obstructions is scheduled for an on-pump coronary artery bypass graft (CABG) but asks the nurse why she is not a candidate for the minimally invasive direct CABG, the most appropriate response is to tell the patient that minimally invasive direct CABG is used only for one-vessel disease in anterior portions of the coronary arteries. With the minimally invasive approach, the incision is made between the ribs but no bones are cut.

76. A: If a patient in minor alcohol withdrawal is prescribed chlordiazepoxide, the purpose of this benzodiazepine is to stabilize the patient's vital signs and to prevent seizures and delirium. The patient may also receive thiamine (vitamin $B_1$) to prevent Wernicke encephalopathy, as alcoholic patients are often deficient in thiamine. If symptoms are severe or seizures occur, then carbamazepine (Tegretol) or phenytoin (Dilantin) may be added as well as an antipsychotic agent, such as haloperidol (Haldol) or chlorpromazine if the benzodiazepine does not relieve psychoses.

77. D: If a Navajo patient tells the CNS that he has "ghost sickness," the most appropriate response is: "How does ghost sickness make you feel?" This response respects the patient's perception of the disease and helps the nurse to understand what symptoms the patient is attributing to the disorder. The Navajo believe that ghost sickness is brought about by evil spirits and that a tribal healer may be able to overcome the spirit. Typical symptoms include weakness, nightmares, fear, and feelings of suffocation.

78. D: If a patient has suspected heart failure, B-type natriuretic peptide (BNP) is the laboratory test that will show the severity of heart failure. This hormone is secreted by ventricular tissues in response to increased volume and pressure in the ventricles, as occurs with heart failure. Normal values should be less than 100 pg/mL. A level of 250 pg/mL (250 ng/L) is consistent with mild heart failure, 375 pg/mL (375 ng/L) with moderate, 650 pg/mL (650 ng/L) with moderately severe, and 800 pg/mL (800 ng/L) with severe.

79. B: If a patient with hypertrophic cardiomyopathy has been prescribed propranolol, the CNS should inform him and his family members that patients taking the drug are at risk of depression, affecting 50% or more, especially those with a history of depression or substance abuse. The patient should be aware of the signs and symptoms of depression and should notify the healthcare provider if they occur. The patient should be advised to never abruptly stop the drug as doing so could cause a myocardial infarction or cardiac arrest.

80. D: If the CNS is examining a patient with circulatory impairment of the lower extremities, the CNS should recognize rubor on dependency and pallor on elevation as indications of arterial insufficiency. Other indications include pain that ranges from intermittent to severe and constant. The skin is often pale and shiny with loss of hair and may feel cool to the touch. Nails may be thickened and ridged. Peripheral pulses are weak or absent but edema is minimal. Ulcerations may occur on the toe tips, toe webs, heels, and other pressure areas, and are often deep, circular, and necrotic.

81. A: If a 50-year-old female patient has symptoms consistent with mitral stenosis, when completing the history and physical exam, the CNS should ask specifically about a history of rheumatic fever because rheumatic fever is the most common cause of mitral stenosis. Mitral stenosis is 4 times more common for females than males, and symptoms often do not occur until the fourth or fifth decade because the valve narrows slowly. Mild mitral stenosis occurs when the vale area is 1 to 1.5 cm² (normal valve area is 4 to 6 cm²).

82. C: If the CNS is using the BVMGR (beliefs, values, meanings, goals, and relationships) rubric for implementing spiritual care, these aspects apply to assessment of the patient. That is, the CNS should try to understand the patient's BVMGR and should not let personal BVMGR intrude and should avoid any indication of proselytizing when the CNS's BVMGR is at odds with the patient's. While the CNS may not share the patient's belief system, the CNS should always seek to understand and to show respect for it.

83. C: When the CNS is assisting a physician with synchronized cardioversion for a patient with unstable atrial fibrillation, before the physician places the paddles, the CNS should check the machine to ensure it is properly sensing R waves. The initial energy level for unstable atrial fibrillation is usually 100 joules. If the cardioversion is unsuccessful, it may be repeated 2 to 3 times at increasing energy levels. If ventricular fibrillation occurs as a result on cardioversion, then the mode is switched from synchronized to defibrillate and the patient is immediately defibrillated.

84. A: If a patient in good health had sudden onset of weakness, chest pain, and dyspnea with systolic BP palpable at 52 mm Hg, pulse 128 bpm, respiratory rate 38 breaths/minute, and oxygen saturation of 81% on room air, then the test that may be used to rule out pulmonary embolism is the D-dimer assay. If the test is negative, then pulmonary embolism is unlikely, but if it is positive, then imaging, such as CT scan or pulmonary angiography, should be carried out. Arterial blood gases, while not diagnostic for pulmonary embolism, should be done to determine the patient's acid-base status.

85. A: If the Richmond Agitation and Sedation Scale (RASS) is used to help titrate sedation for a patient with acute lung injury (ALI) who is intubated and receiving mechanical ventilation, the CNS should ensure that the RASS score is maintained at -1 to -2.

| Less sedated | More sedated |
|---|---|
| +4 combative<br>+3 very agitated<br>+2 agitated<br>+1 restless<br> 0 alert and calm | -5 unarousable<br>-4 deep sedation<br>-3 moderate<br>   sedation<br>-2 light sedation<br>-1 drowsy |

86. B: If a postoperative patient exhibits signs of acute hyponatremia after developing severe nausea and vomiting (confusion, tonic-clonic seizure), and the patient's sodium level at 123 mEq/L (123 mmol/L) is below normal (normal value 135 to 145 mEq/L [135 to 145 mmol/L]) and nearing the critical value of 120 mEq/L (120 mmol/L), and the CNS is to administer 100 mL of 3% NaCl over 10 minutes and to repeat up to 3 times as necessary, the initial goal for increase in the sodium level in the first hour to prevent brain herniation is 4 to 6 mEq/L (4 to 6 mmol/L). Correcting hyponatremia too rapidly can result in osmotic demyelination syndrome (ODS).

87. D: If the CNS is evaluating a patient with a history of aortic insufficiency, the CNS should plan to assess the patient for left-sided heart failure. With aortic insufficiency, blood backflows into the left ventricle during diastole, causing the ventricle to dilate and hypertrophy. Patients often experience exertional dyspnea and paroxysmal nocturnal dyspnea. The patient may also have peripheral edema and ascites. In some cases, a visible apical pulse is noted on inspection of the chest, and the patient's head may bob with each heartbeat.

88. D: A history of diabetes mellitus, major abdominal/thoracic trauma, and neurological disorders increases the risk of aspiration for a patient receiving tube feedings. Patients should be positioned with the head elevated to 45 degrees if possible, and the supine position should be avoided. Continuous feedings pose less risk than intermittent or bolus feedings, and the older patient is at greater risk than the younger. Metoclopramide may be given to increase the rate of gastric emptying. The tube should be checked for correct position at every feeding or every 4 to 6 hours if feedings are continuous.

89. C: The type of aspiration that will produce the most severe pulmonary damage is acid food particles (such as partially digested gastric contents). Patients typically exhibit severe hypoxemia, hypercapnia, and acidosis. The patient's upper airway is usually suctioned to remove as many food particles as possible and may require a bronchoscopy for further removal. The patient's oxygenation and hemodynamics must be supported with supplemental oxygen or mechanical ventilation. Antibiotic therapy is usually initiated in 48 hours if symptoms persist.

90. A: If the CNS is educating a patient with obstructive sleep apnea who is to use a BiPAP machine after discharge, the CNS should stress that the patient must use the BiPAP machine whenever sleeping, even for naps. The patient should be encouraged to establish better sleeping habits, falling asleep at the same time, and avoiding excessive sleeping in the daytime. Many patients with obstructive sleep apnea have slept poorly for years and compensate by napping.

91. B: If a patient with pulmonary arterial hypertension (WHO II) has started treatment with combination therapy that initially includes ambrisentan 5 mg (Letairis) and tadalafil 20 mg (Adcirca) as well as supplementary oxygen for exertion, when educating the patient about disease management, the CNS should tell the patient to be especially alert for signs of peripheral edema, the most common adverse effect. In some cases, pulmonary edema may also occur. Diuretic therapy, such as furosemide, may be added to the regimen. The patient should also have hemoglobin monitored routinely because of increased risk of anemia.

92. C: If an HIV-positive 42-year-old man has developed cytomegalovirus pneumonia, a priority intervention should include ganciclovir (Cytovene) and CMV immune globulin (CMV-IG), which potentiates the action of ganciclovir. CMV infections are usually mild and self-limiting, but if the host is immunocompromised, CMV can result in severe infections throughout the body. The patient must be carefully monitored during treatment as the drug may cause neutropenia, thrombocytopenia, and anemia. Treatment is usually intravenous as oral ganciclovir is less effective.

93. D: If a patient is diagnosed with tuberculosis and must take antituberculosis drugs, taking methadone for heroin addiction may be an indication for directly observed therapy (DOT). With DOT, a healthcare worker administers each dose and observes the patient taking the medication to ensure that the treatment regimen is followed. Other indications include MDR-TB and XDR-TB, sputum cultures positive for acid-fast bacilli, psychiatric disease or cognitive impairment, homelessness, and demonstrated lack of adherence to treatment.

94. D: Adult patients with cystic fibrosis are especially at risk of *Pseudomonas aeruginosa* pneumonia. This type of pneumonia is especially lethal because it causes hemorrhage by invading blood vessels. Outbreaks have occurred in CF clinics. Treatment includes combination of 2 antibiotics (with vancomycin usually avoided because of risk of increase in vancomycin-resistant organisms) and isolation of patients. Preventive measures include using standard precautions, placing patients on mechanical ventilation in 30 degrees upright position, and following protocol for changing ventilator circuits.

95. B: If a patient with latex allergy is inadvertently exposed to latex and develops severe anaphylaxis with difficulty breathing, the priority intervention is to establish an airway and administer epinephrine. The epinephrine should be administered intramuscularly into the vastus lateralis (thigh) muscle instead of the deltoid, as absorption is more rapid. Patients should receive adjunctive therapy with an antihistamine (such as diphenhydramine), corticosteroid (to prevent a biphasic reaction), and an H2 blocker (such as ranitidine).

96. B: If a patient who suffered blunt thoracic trauma exhibits paradoxical movement of the chest during inspiration and expiration with tenderness and crepitation noted on palpation, these findings are consistent with flail chest, which is best confirmed by MSCT scan and arterial blood gases, as hypoxia may be present. Flail chest occurs when 2 or more ribs in 2 or more places are fractured and floating unattached from the thoracic cage. Flail chest is often associated with underlying injury to lung tissue. Chest x-rays may not show all fractures or clearly indicate a pneumothorax.

97. A: If a patient who has had a "sore throat and cough" for the previous 5 days comes to the ED with muffled voice and respiratory distress, appears feverish and cyanotic, and is sitting in tripod position with the mouth open and tongue out, drooling and leaning forward with a heart rate of 112 bpm, the priority intervention should be establishing an airway as these are typical signs of upper airway obstruction, such as from epiglottitis. Arterial blood gases should also be done to assess hypoxia.

98. D: If a patient is brought to the ED with a Glasgow Coma Scale score of 12, the CNS expects the patient to be confused but able to follow simple commands as this score indicates moderate head injury.

| Glasgow Coma Scale | |
|---|---|
| **Eye opening** | 4: spontaneous <br> 3: to verbal stimuli <br> 2: to pain [not of face] <br> 1: no response |
| **Verbal** | 5: oriented <br> 4: conversation confused, but can answer questions <br> 3: uses inappropriate words <br> 2: speech incomprehensible <br> 1: no response |
| **Motor** | 6: moves on command <br> 5: moves purposefully to respond to pain <br> 4: withdraws in response to pain <br> 3: decorticate posturing (flexion) in response to pain <br> 2: decerebrate posturing (extension) in response to pain <br> 1: no response |

Mild = 13 to 15, Moderate = 9 to 12, and Severe = ≤ 8

99. C. Because the normal fasting serum glucose level rules out diabetes mellitus as the cause of the increased thirst and urination and the sodium level is elevated at 152 mEq/L (152 mmol/L), the patient should have serum and urine osmolality tests to determine if the patient has diabetes insipidus, which can result from brain injury or surgery. Diagnostic criteria include:
- Serum sodium: > 145 mEq/L
- Serum osmolality: > 195 mOsm/kg $H_2O$ (> 295 mmol/L)
- Urine osmolality: < 200 mOsm/kg $H_2O$ (< 200 mmol/L)
- Urine specific gravity: < 1.005

100. C: If a patient underwent a right pneumonectomy because of malignant lesions and 6 days after surgery exhibits increasing dyspnea and fever and begins to cough up serosanguineous sputum, and the chest x-rays show sudden increased fluid level in the right pleural space, the CNS should suspect bronchopleural fistula. A bronchopleural fistula occurs when the suture line of the bronchial stump fails and an opening occurs between the bronchial stump and the pleural space. Emergent surgical repair is necessary to prevent the remaining lung from filling with fluid.

101. A: According to the Star Model of systems thinking, if the CNS makes a change in one area of nursing care within an organization, the CNS should expect that this will necessitate a change in another area. The Star Model is based on a diagram with 5 elements (strategy, structure, human resources, incentives, and information/decision-making) that surround core culture and values. In this model, one element is as important as the others, and change in organization culture and values requires indirect action through one of the elements, although ingrained culture and values can stand in the way of progress.

102. C: If the CNS feels that the organization is not receptive to change and wants to use a systems approach to facilitating change, steps include
- Defining the issue: This first step should be done without judgment or solutions.
- Describing patterns of behavior: Factors that relate to the problem.
- Establishing cause and effect relationships. May utilize 5 whys or other root cause analysis.
- Defining patterns of performance/behavior: Relationship of variables and outcomes.
- Finding solutions: Possible solutions to problems and outcomes.
- Instituting performance improvement activities: Make and monitor changes.

103. B: If the CNS needs to delegate a task to an LVN/LPN but is unsure how the nurse performs because the CNS has not worked with this LVN/LPN before, the best initial approach is to ask the LVN/LPN how the person would go about doing the task. Then, the CNS should share expectations and any specific instructions, including under what conditions and when the LVN/LPN needs to report to the CNS and how the CNS will supervise.

104. C: If the CNS notes that staffing patterns do not always match workload, the first step to a solution is to determine how staffing decisions are made. The CNS should always take action based on relevant information and data. The CNS should try to understand the views of management as well as personal and staff views in order to identify areas of agreement and possible compromise before researching staffing alternate methods and making suggestions for change.

105. B: If the CNS notes that one nursing team member often avoids taking care of older patients and sometimes makes disparaging remarks about them, the most appropriate response is for the

CNS to discuss attitudes toward aging with the nurse. People who exhibit ageism are often concerned about their own aging and may be unaware of their bias against older adults. However, the CNS should also make clear that older patients must receive the same quality of care as younger patients and that negative comments about elderly patients are inappropriate.

106. A: Scant tissue loss: Partial thickness injury and ≤ 25% of epidermal flap lost. Payne-Martin classification for skin tears:

| Payne-Martin Classification for Skin Tears | |
|---|---|
| **Category I** Skin tear without tissue loss | -Linear: full-thickness wound in wrinkle or furrow with epidermis and dermis pulled apart (incisional appearance) -Flap: partial thickness wound with a flap that can cover wound with ≤ 1 mm of dermis exposed |
| **Category II** Skin tear with partial tissue loss | -Scant tissue loss: partial thickness injury and ≤ 25% of epidermal flap lost -Moderate-large tissue loss: partial thickness injury with > 25% epidermal flap lost |
| **Category III** Skin tear with complete tissue loss | -Complete partial thickness injury with loss of epidermal flap |

107. C: If the CNS must irrigate an open wound with normal saline as part of routine dressing changes, the psi during irrigation should be no greater than 15 psi because a greater pressure may cause tissue damage, but psi below 4 is inadequate. A bulb syringe produces about 4.5 psi. The pressure varies according to syringe size and needle size if using syringe and needle:

| Syringe mL | Gauge | psi |
|---|---|---|
| 35 | 25 | 4 |
| 35 | 21 | 6 |
| 35 | 19 | 8 |
| 12 | 22 | 13 |
| 12 | 19 | 20 |
| 6 | 19 | 30 |

108. B: If an 80-year-old patient with a history of intraabdominal surgery and diverticulosis has simple incomplete small bowel obstruction (without compromised blood flow) and has had nausea and vomiting for 2 days, the initial interventions that are most indicated are NG decompression and IV fluids (isotonic). The patient will likely also require potassium replacement because hypokalemia is commonly associated with bowel obstruction and vomiting. The most likely cause (and the most common) for the small bowel obstruction is adhesions.

109. D: If the CNS observes a certified nursing assistant (CNA) massaging the reddened heels of an immobile patient, the CNS should explain how massaging reddened tissue may cause tissue damage. This was one time common practice, so the CNS should use this opportunity to update the CNA on evidence-based skin care guidelines and should provide guidance to the CNA regarding measures to relieve pressure, including the use of heel protectors, positioning, and frequent turning.

110. C: If a patient's friend is visiting and expresses concern about the patient and asks for an update on the patient's prognosis, the CNS should tell the visitor the CNS cannot discuss the

patient's condition. Doing so would be a HIPAA violation. The CNS can only discuss a patient's condition with a parent/caregiver of a minor child, a spouse, or a person with the patient's power of attorney without permission from the patient.

111. B: If a patient has suspected kidney disease, the test that will provide the best information about renal function and the glomerular filtration rate (GFR) is the serum creatinine. Serum creatinine levels only increase in the presence of renal impairment, so it is more sensitive than the blood urea nitrogen (BUN), which can also be used to estimate the GFR. The creatinine clearance rate shows how efficiently the kidneys remove creatinine from the blood, so if the serum creatinine increases, the creatinine clearance rate decreases.

112. D: According to systems theory (Bertalanffy), the 5 elements of a system include:
- Input: This is what goes into a system in terms of energy or materials.
- Throughput: These are the actions that take place in order to transform input.
- Output: This is the result of the interrelationship between input and processes.
- Evaluation: Monitoring success or failure.
- Feedback: This is information that results from the process and can be used to evaluate the end result.

113. A: If an 18-year-old patient ingested 10,000 mg of extra-strength acetaminophen and was found by her parents 12 hours later, pale, nauseated, and diaphoretic but without vomiting, the CNS should recognize that the patient is at risk of liver failure. The maximum dose for acetaminophen in 24 hours is 4,000 mg, and severe liver damage can occur at 7,000 mg. The chance for recovery is good if treatment is instituted within 8 hours of ingestion.

114. D: If the hospital administration has collected patient surveys to determine the needs that patients feel are most important, the next step in the quality improvement process should be to assemble a multidisciplinary team to review the results of the survey. Next, the team should collect data about the current status of these needs and determine measurable outcomes and quality indicators. Then, the team should select a plan, implement the plan, and collect data to evaluate outcomes.

115. C: If, as part of clinical inquiry, the CNS is researching evidence-based practice, PubMed is a free abstract database that does not require subscription and contains over 26 million citations for biomedical articles. PubMed includes Medline, which indexes over 5600 medical journals according to subject heading. While PubMed does not provide full-text articles, if these are available, PubMed provides a link. PubMed was developed by the National Center for Biotechnology Information (NCBI) at the US National Library of Medicine (NLM).

116. A: If the CNS is newly hired at a healthcare organization and believes that there is a need for improvement, the first thing the CNS should assess is the workplace culture. The CNS should determine which members of the staff have the most influence over decisions and should determine the values, attitudes, and beliefs of the organization and staff and the degree to which the culture is receptive to change. Immediately proposing changes without first understanding the workplace culture may lead to discord and resistance.

117. B: If the CNS is encouraging team members to use the STAR approach to patient safety, the CNS explains that the STAR approach includes the following steps:

| STAR approach | |
|---|---|
| S | **S**top to concentrate on the task at hand. |
| T | **T**hink about the best way to carry out the task. |
| A | **A**ct to accomplish the necessary task. |
| R | **R**eview the success of or problems with the task completion. |

118. C: If the CNS is concerned that a number of patients have fallen and has convinced the administration to purchase additional lift equipment and assistive devices, the CNS's next step should be to develop safety protocols for lifting/handling patients. The CNS should engage other staff members in this process of developing protocols so that they understand the rationale and benefits, and then train staff members so that they know how to use the equipment and to follow the protocols.

119. C: If the CNS notes that a patient's BP has fallen precipitously and the pulse rate has increased but fails to inform the patient's physician and the patient suffers permanent injury as a result, the element of malpractice that applies to the CNS is breach of duty owed. Duty owed to the patient is usually established by employment records or agreements to provide care, and breach of duty owed to the patient occurs when a nurse who has a duty to care for a patient provides care that is below standard.

120. D: Minors may give valid informed consent under only a few circumstances, including those who have been granted emancipation by the courts. The age of adult status is determined by the state and is generally 18. However, adult status is conferred on those who are legally married, regardless of age. In most states, minors can give informed consent for treatment for STDs, pregnancy, and substance abuse. Laws regarding the right to consent to abortion vary from state to state.

121. A: If 2 members of the CNS's team have become embroiled in a conflict, an example of the defensive mode of conflict management would be if the CNS assigned the 2 members to different schedules. The defensive mode usually does not serve to solve the conflict but rather to avoid it. Compromise and problem solving are more effective, but if these fail, the defensive mode may be the only way to manage the destructiveness of the conflict.

122. B: If the CNS discovers that a patient faces various problems in returning home after discharge, including lack of adequate income and impaired ability to prepare food, and refers the patient to a social worker for assistance, the type of power that the CNS is exhibiting is advocacy power because the CNS is assisting the patient to overcome obstacles. Integrative power helps the patient return to normal life. Transformational power helps patients transform their self-image. Affirmative power is the strength the CNS gains from caring for patients. Advocacy power is removing obstacles.

123. A: Generally, the cultural context of a patient from Russia would be considered *low* context, that is the meaning comes from the explicit spoken or written words, as opposed to *high* context, where the meaning derives from the situation itself (context) and much is omitted from words. People from cultures with low context (including most Americans) tend to be more verbal in describing problems or concerns and have more concern for the individual as opposed to the group.

124. D: When working with a diverse group of staff members, the CNS should recognize that the generational group that is most likely to look at duty in terms of personal needs, enjoy teamwork, and expect positive feedback despite the level of performance is the Millennials (also called Generation Y). This group was born between about 1980 and 2000, and its members have grown up as part of the digital world, often preferring information in small "bites."

125. B: Considering the elements of a system and how it relates to health care, nursing services provided by the CNS would be considered part of throughputs. System elements include:
- Inputs: money, individuals, technology, resources
- Throughputs: processes and interactions, including nursing services
- Outputs: clinical outcomes
- Feedback: accreditation, regulations, malpractice suits, patient satisfaction, staff satisfaction

126. A: If the CNS is in a management position and is basing management strategies on the contingency theory, the leadership style that the CNS would utilize would be dependent on the situation. For example, in an emergency situation, the autocratic style of management may be more effective and allow for rapid decision making, while for other concerns, a more democratic or consultative management style may produce better results.

127. C: If the CNS has instituted staff rounding with the goal of meeting with each staff member at least once weekly, the purpose of staff rounding is to improve communication and support staff member's needs. Typical questions include asking about what's working well, who should be recognized for good work, what needs improved, whether the staff member has needed tools, and equipment, and whether the person needs help. The overall goal is to improve staff satisfaction and reduce turnover.

128. D: If the CNS wants to initiate a process of change in an organization, the CNS must realize that the first essential element of the change process is the belief in the possibility of change. Without this belief, staff members are not willing to put forth effort that they feel will be for nothing. Once the belief is present, then a decision can be made and actions taken to lead to change. The results of change should be evaluated, as this helps lead to an understanding of the entire change process.

129. A: If, when reviewing staffing needs, the CNS finds that staff members' time is most impacted by answering patients' call lights and responding to their needs, the strategy that is likely to be most effective for time saving is rounding on patients hourly. Rounding involves actually visiting each patient briefly to ask about and attend to needs, such as for pain control or toileting. Studies indicate that hourly rounding decreases call lights, falls, and pressure sores, and increases patient satisfaction.

130. C: If an organization has instituted Individualized Patient Care and one of the patients tells the CNS that his idea of excellent care is "to be left in peace and quiet," the CNS should clarify what the patient means. It is possible the patient simply wants to take a nap or is expressing grief about being ill through anger or withdrawal, but the patient may also need to express feelings, and this presents an opportunity to encourage the patient to do so.

131. B: If a patient is diagnosed with a non-Q-wave myocardial infarction, the CNS should anticipate that reperfusion will occur spontaneously because the MI is rarely transmural and the infarction is usually small in size, with coronary occlusion occurring in only 20% to 30%. The ECG is characterized by ST depression. While mortality rates are only 2% to 3%, reinfarction frequently

occurs. Peak creatine kinase (CK) levels occur in about 12 to 13 hours (compared with 27 hours for Q-wave MIs).

132. D: If a patient with immune thrombocytopenic purpura (ITP) has a platelet count of 70,000/mm³ and is scheduled for a breast biopsy, and the CNS notifies the surgeon about the level, the CNS should expect the biopsy to be carried out with further treatment. While normal values range from 150,000 to 450,000/mm³, the critical value at which the risk of bleeding may occur is 50,000/mm³ but complex surgeries, such as cardiac surgery, may best be done at 100,000/mm³. Minor procedures may often safely be done at levels of 20,000 to 30,000/mm³.

133. C: If a patient who developed polyarthralgia was recently diagnosed with systemic lupus erythematosus, when educating the patient about lifestyle changes, the CNS should plan to include energy conservation and skin protection. Fatigue is a chronic problem, so the patient must learn to pace activities and schedule periods of rest. Patients must ensure skin integrity by avoiding exposure to the sun, inspecting skin routinely, and using sunscreens. Patients also require education regarding management of chronic pain through analgesic and non-analgesic means.

134. B: The CNS should advise a patient who has had a gastrectomy to be monitored routinely for anemia. Patients are especially at risk of pernicious anemia because of a lack of or inadequate supply of intrinsic factor so that vitamin $B_{12}$ is not adequately absorbed. The decrease in gastric acid, which is needed to promote absorption of dietary iron by the intestines, can result in iron deficiency anemia as well. Patients should also be advised of increased risk of osteoporosis because of impaired calcium absorption.

135. C: If the CNS has taught a patient's spouse to change the patient's dressing and to understand signs of both healing and infection, the best method to ensure that the patient's spouse is able to carry out the dressing change and monitor the wound is to ask for a return demonstration. The CNS should ask the spouse to change the dressing while the CNS observes and to "talk through" the steps during the procedure, including a description of the wound.

136. A: If an 18-year-old football player experienced blunt trauma to his left lower leg during a tackle and was able to walk initially with no difficulty but comes to the hospital about an hour later with severe pain and tightness in the lower leg, a sensation of burning, and the lower leg is edematous and skin taut, although distal pulse is palpable and capillary refill time is within normal limits, the priority intervention should be to measure compartment pressure to confirm compartment syndrome. Distal pulses and capillary refill time may remain intact until the damage is irreversible.

137. B: If a 32-year-old patient suffered carbon monoxide (CO) toxicity and is receiving 100% oxygen per nonrebreather mask, the patient should be maintained on 100% oxygen therapy until she is asymptomatic and the hemoglobin CO level falls to below 10%. If the initial level was above 15%, the patient should be evaluated for cardiovascular complications. Patients with level of greater than 40% and pregnant patients with levels greater than 15% should be referred for hyperbaric treatment.

138. A: If an 80-year-old female patient who developed a urinary tract infection now has a temperature of 39°C (102.2°F), heart rate of 108 bpm, respiration rate 26 breaths/minute, and white blood count of 15,000 with 12% band with blood cultures pending, the CNS would classify the patient's stage of infection as systemic inflammatory response syndrome (SIRS). The condition is reclassified as sepsis when confirmed by culture. Severe sepsis is a progression with organ

dysfunction, hypotension, or hypoperfusion, and septic shock includes both hypotension (despite resuscitation efforts) plus hypoperfusion. Multiorgan dysfunction syndrome (MODS) is progressive failure of 2 or more organ systems.

139. D: If a 73-year-old patient has a 6 cm by 4 cm coccygeal pressure ulcer that extends to the muscle and is partially covered with black necrotic tissue, the CNS would classify the pressure ulcer as stage IV. Stages:

| NPUAP Pressure Ulcer Classification | |
|---|---|
| Suspected | Blood blister, discolored skin, pain, texture change, or temperature change. |
| Stage I | Localized non-blanching reddened area. |
| Stage II | Partial thickness skin los involving epidermis and dermis; abrasion/blistered appearance. |
| Stage III | Exposure of subcutaneous tissue, but not of muscle or bone. |
| Stage IV | Extends to muscle, bone, tendons, or joints with extensive damage and necrosis. |
| Unstageable | Slough and/or eschar in wound makes staging impossible until debridement. |

140. D: If a patient involved in a motorcycle accident fractured the right tibia and fibula, has a new plaster case that is still damp, and says that the cast feels "hot," the CNS should understand that this likely indicates normal sensation from the heat radiating from the skin. The patient should be cautioned to keep the cast uncovered during the drying process so that air can circulate. The patient should be turned at least every 2 hours so that new areas of the cast are exposed and the cast dries evenly.

141. A: If the CNS intends to implement a new procedure in the delivery of patient care, the CNS should understand that the biggest threat to implementation of change is usually staff resistance. For this reason, it is important for the CNS to obtain "buy in" as part of preparation and to identify and recruit key individuals who are likely to influence others to promote change. Staff resistance can be passive (lack of enthusiasm, complaining) or active (refusing to participate, undermining efforts).

142. D: Performing. The 4 stages of team development include:
1) Forming: Leader is most active. Characteristics include anxiety, testing, and excitement.
2) Storming: Opinions begin to diverge. Characteristics include stress, resistance, and competitiveness.
3) Norming: Members feel positive toward each other and identify with the group. Characteristics include satisfaction, trust, mutual respect, and shared decision making.
4) Performing: Leader's role decreases. Characteristics include optimism and confidence.
5) Mourning: Members feel sad when group process ends or members leave the group.

143. C: If the CNS comes to work early to see a patient who reminds her of her mother, brings the patient small gifts, and is judgmental about the patient's family members' actions, the CNS is exhibiting the countertransference reaction of over-involvement. Countertransference is the inappropriate (and often unconscious) transfer of feelings and behaviors from a person in the CNS's life onto a patient. Countertransference interferes with the therapeutic relationship and disempowers the patient.

144. D: If a patient with osteomyelitis has not responded adequately to IV antibiotics and is to continue with oral ciprofloxacin after discharge, and the patient asks the CNS how progress toward healing will be monitored, the CNS should advise the patient that osteomyelitis is usually monitored with periodic bone scans (such as CT scans) or MRI and the erythrocyte sedimentation rate (ESR). Bone x-rays will not show the extent of soft tissue involvement.

145. B: If a patient has a temporary external transcutaneous pacemaker in place for bradycardia and the CNS has adjusted the pacemaker rate setting and identified the pacing threshold, the output setting should be set at 2 to 3 times the measured threshold because thresholds often vary over time. When determining the pacing threshold, the CNS should begin by increasing the rate setting so that the patient is 100% paced and then decreasing the setting until capture is lost and increasing slowly again until recapture occurs.

146. D: If the CNS is caring for a patient with kidney failure and a falling GFR of 28 mL/min/1.73 m², the CNS should recognize that the patient is at stage 3 and will need renal replacement therapy when the GFR is less than 15 ml/min/1.73 m². Stages:
1) GFR > 90 mL/min/1.73 m². Usually asymptomatic.
2) GFR 60 to 89 mL/min/1.73 m². Mild anemia/electrolyte imbalances.
3) GFR 30 to 59 mL/min/1.73 m². Increasing fatigue, anemia, fluid retention, and blood pressure.
4) GFR 15 to 29 mL/min/1.73 m². Profound disease.
5) GFR < 15 mL/min/1.73 m². Kidney failure.

147. A: If a patient with a history of aggression begins swearing and pacing back and forth, yelling, "You can't make me stay here!" the best initial response from the CNS is to speak calmly and quietly to the patient. The CNS should remain in control and avoid reactions that suggest fear or anger. The nurse should stand if sitting but avoid moving aggressively toward the patient but should move toward the door if the situation appears to be escalating and it is safe to do so.

148. B: If the CNS is monitoring the waveform during insertion of a pulmonary artery catheter and observes the waveform in the graphic, the CNS should recognize it as the right ventricular waveform. The first visible waveform during insertion is the right atrial waveform, indicating the catheter has advanced into the right atrium. This is followed by the right ventricular waveform and then the pulmonary artery waveform. Once the balloon in inflated in the pulmonary artery and advanced to wedge position, the pulmonary artery occlusion waveform should be evident.

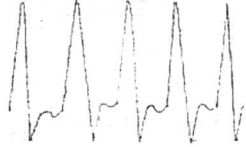

149. D: A patient who reports having the "flu" with 3 days of nausea, vomiting, diarrhea with watery stools, and inability to eat or drink anything excepts sips of ginger ale has vital signs of BP 106/82 mm Hg, pulse rate of 90 bpm, respiratory rate of 24 breaths/minute, urine specific gravity of 1.036, serum sodium 152 mEq/L (152 mmol/L), and serum potassium of 3.1 mEq/L (3.1 mmol/L). The patient's priority treatment is for IV fluids for deficient fluid volume and potassium for hypokalemia. Deficient fluid volume is consistent with hypernatremia (normal value 135 to 145 mEq/L) and increased specific gravity (normal value 1.005 to 1.03). Hypokalemia (normal value 3.5 to 5.3 mEq/L) requires treatment to prevent cardiac abnormalities.

150. C: If a patient with Guillain-Barré syndrome is hospitalized and placed on mechanical ventilation because of ascending paralysis and increasing dyspnea, the priority intervention should be high-dose immunoglobulin. The immunoglobulin helps to fight the infection. An alternate treatment is plasmapheresis, which is more complicated but equally effective. No advantage has been found from using both treatments. With severe paralysis, patients may require mechanical ventilation until paralysis recedes and may have permanent neurological impairment. Steroids may worsen the condition, and antibiotics and antivirals are ineffective.

151. B: If the CNS overhears another nurse complaining that an adult female Hmong patient is subservient and dependent because she allows her father to make decisions about her health care and that the nurse tried without success to convince the patient to make her own decisions, this type of intervention would *best* be described as cultural imposition. The nurse is trying to impose a cultural norm that is different from that of the patient. In the Hmong community, the eldest male in the family is usually the one to make decisions, and this is a respected tradition.

152. A: When the CNS is assessing a patient with neurological injury, an upper motor neuron lesion is indicated by muscle spasticity. Other indications include hyperactive reflexes, loss of voluntary muscle control, and increased muscle tone but no evidence of muscle atrophy. However, with a lower motor neuron lesion, while the patient also lacks voluntary muscle control, decreased muscle tone and muscle flaccidity as well as decreased or absent reflexes and atrophy of muscles are also exhibited.

153. D: If a patient who experienced tonic-clonic seizures is newly diagnosed with epilepsy and has started antiseizure medication, when the CNS is educating the patient about the disease, the most important advice is to never stop taking the medication abruptly as this can trigger status epilepticus, which is life-threatening. The patient should be advised to consult the physician if unable to take medication for any reason, such as illness. The patient should exercise in moderation, avoid excessive heat, and try to distinguish triggers and auras related to seizures to better manage the disorder.

154. C: If the CNS is working the night shift and finds it increasingly difficult to stay awake during the night, the best way to ensure the CNS is alert during the night is to sleep immediately before beginning the night shift. If it is not possible to schedule a long period of sleep at this time, then the CNS should try to nap for at least 2 hours before going to work. Lack of sleep and tiredness are safety issues because the CNS may have impaired cognition as a result of fatigue.

155. B: If a 25-year-old patient's BMI is 17.5 (normal 18.5 to 24.9), the patient is underweight and likely lacks adequate caloric intake. The patient's albumin level is within normal limits at 3.8 g/dL (38 g/L), reflecting adequate long-term protein intake; however, the prealbumin level is low at 6 mg/dL (60 mg/L) (normal 16 to 40 mg/dL [160 to 400 mg/L]). Prealbumin has a half-life of 2 to 3 days (compared with 18 to 20 for albumin), so it reflects acute (short-term) protein malnutrition.

156. A: If a patient with acute appendicitis awaiting surgery has pain despite analgesia, the position that may help to alleviate discomfort is bending the right knee to relieve tension on the abdominal muscles. However, if the knee is elevated against pressure, this causes tensing of the psoas muscle that is near the appendix and increases pain. Heating pads should be avoided as they may increase the risk of rupture of the appendix.

157. D: Confirmability. In evaluating research as part of the development of evidence-based practice guidelines, the 4 evaluative/trustworthiness criteria are:
- Credibility: Documentation supports accuracy and validity.
- Dependability: Evidence shows how conclusion are reached and whether others should expect to each the same conclusions.
- Transferability: The extent to which the results can apply to others in similar situations.
- Confirmability: The data are clear and show how conclusions are reached.

158. B: If a patient who works in a daycare center and handles food is diagnosed with hepatitis A after developing flu-like symptoms, the patient was likely contagious for 2 weeks prior to onset of symptoms. The patient may remain contagious for 1 to 2 weeks after onset as well. Hepatitis A is primarily spread through the fecal-oral route, although the virus is present in the blood for a short period of time.

159. C: A 66-year-old male patient has increasing abdominal pain and has been passing 3 to 4 sticky, black, foul-smelling stools for 3 to 4 days. His vital signs are 116/78 mm Hg supine, pulse rate 112 bpm, respiratory rate 22 breaths/minute, and temperature 37°C (98.6°F), while standing BP dropped to 88/58 mm Hg with dizziness, and hemoglobin is 9.2 mg/dL (92 mmol/L), hematocrit 28%, mean corpuscular volume (MCV) 90 fL, and BUN 46 mg/dL (16.4 mmol/L), the CNS should suspect iron deficiency anemia with upper GI bleeding. The anemia occurs from blood loss (low hemoglobin and hematocrit with normal MCV) and the melena is from blood in the upper GI tract that is exposed to digestive enzymes. The elevated BUN reflects absorption of blood.

160. A: If a patient with multiple sclerosis tells the nurse that she is upset that she can no longer continue her employment because her job is too physically demanding and is concerned about how she will support herself, the response that focuses on problem solving as a response to stress is, "What plans do you have for finding a new job?" This response does not suggest a solution, such as public assistance, but indirectly suggests that the patient can take control to solve the problem.

161. D: If a patient recently returned from serving in the military in the Middle East is hospitalized with post-traumatic stress disorder and has recurring flashbacks and nightmares and is constantly vigilant and anxious, telling the CNS repeatedly that he should have died with his friends, the most appropriate response is, "Are you thinking about killing yourself?" When a patient gives clues about suicidal ideation, it is the CNS's responsibility to address the issue with the patient, and patients often want to talk about their feelings.

162. B: If the CNS is screening patients for referral to a case manager, the patient that is most likely to benefit from case management is the 62-year-old patient with repeated hospitalizations from COPD and diabetes. Criteria for case management include patients with severe chronic illness and comorbidities, especially those with a history of repeated hospitalizations or noncompliance with treatment and those who are elderly, disabled, or impaired and lack an adequate support system.

163. C: If the CNS is supervising a novice nurse, the action by the nurse that should cause the CNS to intervene is if the nurse administers medications without checking patient IDs. The nurse must check 2 forms of identification (such as by asking the name or birthdate and verifying the ID name and number) every time medication or treatment is administered even if the nurse is familiar with the patient. The purpose is to ensure that the correct medication/treatment is being administered to the correct patient.

164. D: When the CNS is researching evidence-based practice, the research design that provides the best information about cause and effect relationships is one that utilizes randomized controlled trials (RCT). Randomized controlled trials are designs used in quantitative research. A systematic review of multiple RCTs that have homogeneity (agreement) is the strongest evidence that an intervention will bring about positive and expected outcomes. When researching, the CNS must consider both the clinical significance of the findings and statistical significance.

165. A: If the CNS is teaching a patient with amyotrophic lateral sclerosis (ALS) to manage the disease, an example of the CNS using the tool of *negotiating* is when the CNS presents the pros and cons of treatment. The purpose of negotiating is to help the patient to choose the best course of action through provision of information and clear explanations while respecting the wishes and needs of the patient. Other tools the CNS can utilize include *coaching* (helping patients obtain information needed to manage their own care) and *motivating* (using strategies, such as motivational interviewing to encourage participation).

166. B: If the CNS is preparing patient education materials as part of a series of health classes being offered to patients with chronic illness, when developing instructional materials, the 3 major components that the CNS must consider are the:
- Delivery system: paper, computer, audio, visual, PowerPoint, video
- Content: Information that is to be communicated.
- Presentation: The manner in which the information is presented, from concrete (realia) to abstract (symbolic representation).

167. C: If the CNS has proposed use of the SBAR (Situation-Background-Assessment-Recommendation) format for hand-off communication but is encountering resistance from long-time staff members who dislike change, the best method of dealing with resistance is to encourage staff members to express opinions and discuss concerns. The CNS should answer any questions, provide evidence of benefit, and respond to misperceptions. When change is evidence based and in the best interests of patients, leadership may require change without voting.

168. A: If the CNS is giving an interview to a reporter of a local newspaper about a community health prevention program that the CNS is spearheading, the CNS should avoid scientific jargon and define any medical terms as they occur rather than waiting for the reporter to ask for definitions. The CNS should not suggest a story angle or ask for a prepublication, and should discuss positive aspects of the program but should also include any negative aspects or concerns.

169. B: If a patient with dilated cardiomyopathy is on the transplant list for a heart but none has become available, the patient's ejection fraction has fallen to 22%, and the patient's functional ability is markedly decreased, the CNS should recognize that the patient may benefit most from a left ventricular assist device (LVAD). The LVAD is usually implanted in patients whose ejection fraction is below 25% (normal values range from 55% to 65%). The LVAD augments the heart's ability to pump blood and can be used as a bridge to transplant or as destination treatment for those who are not candidates for transplant.

170. C: If, when analyzing data as part of clinical research, the CNS includes only those cases that relate specifically to the requirement of the measurement and exclude cases that are similar but associated with a different population in order to decrease the number of false-positives, the issue that the CNS is addressing is specificity. Sensitivity requires data that incude all positive cases. Reliability requires that results be reproducible. Validity means that the results can be used to predict because the data and results measure the target adequately.

171. D: According to NANDA guidelines, an example of a problem-focused nursing diagnosis is: Pain related to abdominal incision with inflammation (erythema, edema) as evidenced by verbalization of pain, guarding, and social withdrawal. This is a 3-part nursing diagnosis that follows the PES format: **P**roblem, **E**tiology, and **S**igns and symptoms. Examples of risk-focused diagnoses are: Risk for aspiration as evidenced by dysphagia and impaired cough reflex AND Risk for DVT as evidenced by immobility and peripheral edema. An example of a health promotion nursing diagnosis is: Readiness for discharge as evidenced by independence in self-care.

172. A: If a patient with chronic low back pain states he wants to try complementary therapy to relive pain because medications have been ineffective and asks the CNS which of the therapies are likely to relieve discomfort, the CNS should reply that the therapy that has documented effectiveness is acupuncture. Acupuncture appears to stimulate the production of endorphins. Acupuncture is generally safe and has no adverse effects if done by an experienced practitioner. There is little discomfort involved in treatment.

173. C: The most important factor in determining whether an event is a stressor to a patient is the patient's perception. For example, if 2 patients have kidneys removed for cancer and both are stage I, one patient may be relieved that the stage is low and feel very positive about recovery while the second patient may be overwhelmed with anxiety and fear at the thought of any cancer and may obsess over the possibility of recurrence.

174. C: If a CNS was exposed to tuberculosis at work and developed active pulmonary TB, the CNS must be excluded from work until treatment is completed OR 3 sputum tests are negative. Most work-related cases result from delayed diagnosis of infected patients. When a healthcare worker becomes infected, all those at risk (including nurses, physicians, therapists, volunteers, and housekeeping staff) must be tested as well as patients to whom infected staff members may have passed the infection.

175. A: If the CNS hears a patient's physician complaining that a patient is "difficult and impatient," and the CNS tells the physician that the patient is very frightened and acting defensively, the aspect of care that the nurse is exhibiting is advocacy. The nurse is speaking up in defense of the patient and acting for the patient's benefit in trying to help the physician have a more balanced view of the patient's behavior.